Rabah Kouadria
Ismail Si Ali
Soumia Benbernou

Surgery for intramedullary tumors

Rabah Kouadria
Ismail Si Ali
Soumia Benbernou

Surgery for intramedullary tumors

ScienciaScripts

Imprint
Any brand names and product names mentioned in this book are subject to trademark, brand or patent protection and are trademarks or registered trademarks of their respective holders. The use of brand names, product names, common names, trade names, product descriptions etc. even without a particular marking in this work is in no way to be construed to mean that such names may be regarded as unrestricted in respect of trademark and brand protection legislation and could thus be used by anyone.

Cover image: www.ingimage.com

This book is a translation from the original published under ISBN 978-620-6-71250-3.

Publisher:
Sciencia Scripts
is a trademark of
Dodo Books Indian Ocean Ltd. and OmniScriptum S.R.L publishing group

120 High Road, East Finchley, London, N2 9ED, United Kingdom
Str. Armeneasca 28/1, office 1, Chisinau MD-2012, Republic of Moldova, Europe
Printed at: see last page
ISBN: 978-620-7-63761-4

Rabah KOUADRIA

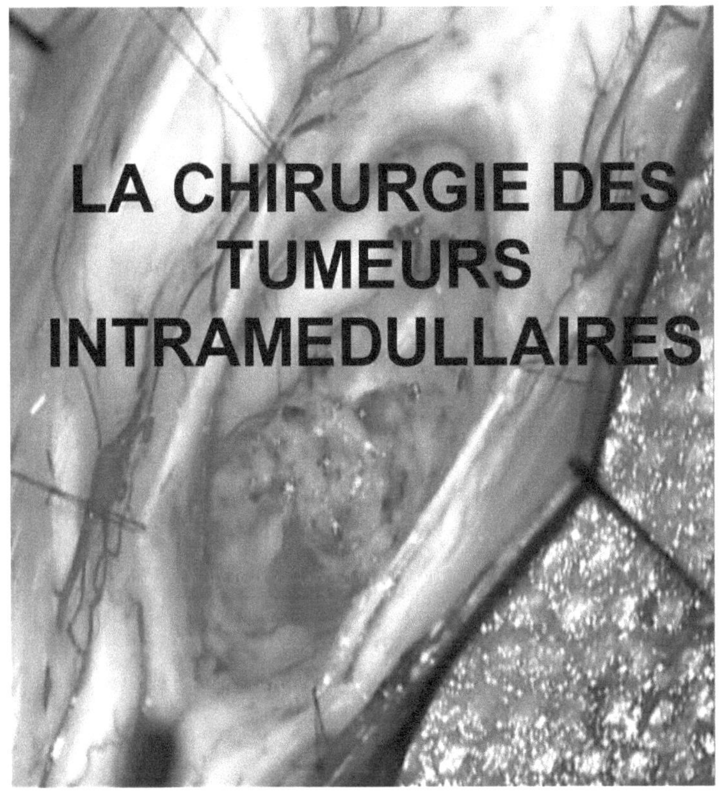

Table of contents

I. INTRODUCTION

Intramedullary tumors (IMT) are a rare pathological entity among tumors of the central nervous system. Surgery for intramedullary tumors has been revolutionized since the introduction of magnetic resonance imaging (MRI) and the operating microscope. Despite these advances in both diagnostic and surgical techniques, surgery remains a major challenge, due to the rarity of IMTs and the consequent lack of accumulated experience. This book is aimed at healthcare professionals involved in the management of spinal cord tumors in general, and IMTs in particular. Its aim is above all to provide an anatomical basis and a diagnostic and therapeutic approach. As a neurosurgeon who has had the privilege of operating almost continuously on patients with spinal cord tumors for almost 17 years, I feel obliged to pass on and share my personal experience and modest contribution to the planning and execution of these surgical procedures, and to make them available to the future generation of neurosurgeons who will surely continue to carry the torch of MCT surgery.

Although treatment is essentially surgical, collaboration with other specialties, including neuroradiologists, neuropathologists, medical and radiation oncologists, neurologists, rehabilitation specialists and other professionals, remains essential to provide patients with the best possible care.

Intramedullary tumors are most often low-grade. They pose considerable diagnostic and management challenges.

The insidious onset and slow progression of symptoms make early diagnosis difficult.

MRI is generally the examination of choice for diagnosing IMT, while CT is rarely used. However, it can never replace histological studies, which can only be carried out through surgery. The latter must allow for a wide and at the same time safe exeresis. The timing and quality of excision is controversial, as early intervention at a paucisymptomatic stage could lead to neurological worsening, while waiting for the onset of deficits can make recovery after excision risky, as can the quality of excision; wide excision will expose the patient to the risk of deficits, while partial excision to recurrence and unpredictable decline.

But more recent, cutting-edge techniques and instruments, such as new imaging modalities, peroperative neurophysiological monitoring and high-quality microscopes, make it easier to distinguish between tumor and healthy tissue, enabling neurosurgeons to reach tumors once considered inaccessible, and to abandon the previous pessimistic conservative approach in favor of an aggressive surgical approach.

Some small tumors that are discovered incidentally or are asymptomatic and show little progression can simply be carefully monitored clinically and with serial MRI at appropriate intervals.

Even with the latest advances in surgical technology, some tumors remain inoperable, and it is sometimes advisable to perform a partial exeresis. In such cases, and depending on the histological nature of the tumor, adjuvant therapy is proposed, i.e. radiotherapy and/or chemotherapy.

Recovery from surgery can take weeks or longer. But the worst thing is the post-operative aggravation, which is fortunately temporary in most cases.

Although corticosteroids reduce inflammation, they are generally only used for short periods to avoid serious side effects such as muscle weakness, osteoporosis, high blood pressure, diabetes and increased susceptibility to infection.

In my short career, I've always tried to make up for my shortcomings and overcome the complications and failures I've had to incur with my respected patients, whose acceptance has been very difficult, especially when it comes to benign tumors. I've learned far more from my complications than from my surgical successes.

We hope that this book will contribute to the development of neurosurgery in general and spinal cord surgery in particular.

II. HISTORY

From the rather primitive beginnings of neurosurgery with Victor Horsley to the current state of the art, IMT surgery has evolved enormously, benefiting from advances in neurosurgery in general and the clinical and scientific contributions of some bold pioneers.

1. THE BEGINNINGS: APPROACHING AND EXERTISING TIMBRES

The first successful excision of a TIM was performed in 1907 in Vienna by Anton Von Eiselsberg on his 27-year-old patient, who had a favourable post-operative outcome [134].

Among the various reports from the end of the first decade of the $20^{\text{ème}}$ century, the work of Charles A. Elsberg stands out. Elsberg, who operated on 2 patients in 1910. In the first, Elsberg and his assistant Edwin accidentally nicked the posterior cord in 2 places; on closer inspection, Elsberg noticed an exit of abnormal tissue through the myelotomy. He rejoined the two openings and lengthened the myelotomy to complete a tumor excision that would instead be stopped due to hemodynamic instability. Elsberg observed that the tumor mass had exited spontaneously, facilitating dissection with the medullary tissue. The patient progressed well and continued to improve. The second case, the opposite of the first, was operated on in a single operation and died a few hours later of respiratory distress. Post-mortem examination revealed no spinal cord injury or haematoma. Elsberg attributed these complications to a more aggressive dissection, so he concluded that this operation would have been safer if performed in two stages, hence the birth of "two-stage surgery" [229]. His 1916 book *Diagnosis and Treatment of Surgical Diseases of the Spinal Cord and*

Its Membranes was highly influential at the time, and remains an impressive document to this day. The two-stage operation is still used today in certain circumstances [103-106].

2. TECHNICAL ADVANCES

In the late 1930s, James Greenwood began using a "two-clamp punctal coagulation" technique developed by Leonard Malis and eventually became what is now known as bipolar coagulation [31]. In 1954, Greenwood [91] published the first series of TIM excisions with long-term follow-up.

In 1948, Carl Zeiss and Ernst were the first to introduce microscopes with high-quality lenses. In 1957, Theodore Kurtz was the first neurosurgeon to use an operating microscope, and trained many neurosurgeons in its use, including Robert Rand, Lawrence Pool and Charles Drake [140].

In 1976, M. Gazi Yasargile and Hugo Krayenbühl [268] published the first microsurgical series of 12 intramedullary hemangioblastomas.

Ultrasonic suction came into medical use in 1947. Originally developed for dental plaque removal, it was put to use in neurosurgery 30 years after its creation by Flamm et al [80]. Shortly afterwards, in 1982, Epstein [74] published an article on its use in IMT surgery.

The recording of somato-sensory evoked potentials began in 1947 with Dawson [229], followed in 1978 by the first publication on somaesthetic evoked potentials (SEPs) in spinal surgery [68]. In the 1980s, a wave of work on motor evoked potentials (MEPs) was published, notably in scoliosis surgery [25]. In 1989, Zentner [273] noted in his report of 50 spinal cord surgeries monitored by MEPs that permanent postoperative neurological deficits coincided with a reduction in baseline amplitudes of more than 50% in each case.

The use of laser scalpels in neurosurgery was initially reported in experimental studies on rabbits [13]. In 1966, Rosomoff et al [215] were the first to report the use of a ruby laser for brain tumor surgery. In 2002, Jallo [119] published the first report on the clinical use of the contact-mode Nd YAG laser as a surgical scalpel for IMT.

3. IMAGERY

In order to visualize the spinal cord and roots, the technique devised in conventional radiology was to inject a contrast medium into the sub-arachnoid spaces to perform myelography.

In the 1950s-1970s, the first radiopaque substances were highly toxic to the central nervous system.

In 1970, Amipaque revolutionized the practice due to its better quality and tolerability, and since then, several increasingly less harmful products have appeared on the market. Since the advent of the CT scanner, and especially the use of sagittal reconstructions coupled with "myeloscanner" opacification of the subarachnoid spaces, this study has lost some of its interest.

In the late 1980s, MRI supplanted both examinations.

3.2. The advent of MRI

The invention of MRI is attributed to Nobel Prize winners who helped discover the behavior of atoms in magnetic fields. In 1977,

Damadian [56] performed MRI of the whole human body; in parallel, Mansfield [163] developed the *Echo-planar imaging* protocol, which enables T2*-weighted images to be acquired much more rapidly than before. In 1983, Norman et al [188] reported on their preliminary experiments with spinal cord MRI in 17 cases.

3.1. Intraoperative ultrasound

Ultrasound was first introduced into neurosurgery by Reid in 1978 [210]. Since the early 1990s, it has been used consistently by Epstein et al. in IMT resection [74].

III. ANATOMICAL OVERVIEW

This anatomical review is a non-exhaustive section of our work, designed to remind us of some basic notions about the spinal cord, its vascularization and its osteomeningeal envelopes.

1. RACHIS

The surgical approach to the spinal cord cannot be conceived without a perfect knowledge of the container represented by the spine and its ligaments.

1.1. Cervical spine

The cervical spine is made up of two "specific" vertebrae: the atlas and the axis, linking the spine to the occiput in a complex set of joints and ligaments, and five "ordinary" vertebrae in a slightly lordotic curve.

In young adults, the average length of the cervical spine is 12.5 cm (11.5 cm in retroflexion and 12.69 cm in anteflexion) [133-163].

The atlas is shaped like a ring, articulating with the occipital condyles above and the axis articularis below via two small lateral masses. A fifth joint, ensuring head rotation, is formed between the atlas and the odontoid. The axis articulates with the lateral masses of C1 above and supports the odontoid in the middle (Figs. 1 and 2).

The rest of the vertebral bodies are rectangular in shape, with a slight depression of the upper surface giving rise to bony ridges on either side known as "uncus".

The posterior elements of the second to seventh vertebrae form the neural arches, which are composed of pedicles, laminae and spinous processes. The short pedicles connect the vertebral bodies to the superior and inferior articular joints. The foramen of conjugation, which is oriented outwards and forwards by 30°, is delimited by the pedicles above and below, the uncus medially, the transverse process laterally and the articular processes posteriorly. The blades project posteriorly to meet the base of the spinous processes. The spinous process tapers posteriorly and inferiorly on the median line. There are no spinous processes in C1, but large spinous processes in C2 and C7. The mean anteroposterior diameter of the bony spinal canal is 18-20 mm in C1 and C2, and 1517 mm between C3 and C7. The dural sac measures 10-14 mm throughout the cervical spine and the spinal cord is 6-9 mm, in other words the spinal cord normally occupies only around 40-50% of the spinal canal.

The medial atlantoaxial joint is stabilized by a complex set of ligaments, the most important of which is the cruciate ligament (vertical and horizontal arms), which lies immediately behind the odontoid in the frontal plane. The horizontal arm, or transverse ligament, is stretched between the lateral masses of C1 and the posterior surface of the odontoid, pressing firmly against the anterior arch of C1. The vertical arm lies between the anterior edge of the foramen magnum and the body of C2 (Figs. 2, 3 and 4).

The odontoid is linked to the skull base by the apical ligament, which extends from its anterior end to the foramen magnum, and the alar ligaments laterally to the occipital condyles. The vertebral bodies are connected by the anterior and posterior longitudinal ligaments from C1 to the sacrum. The anterior longitudinal ligament terminates in the anterior atlanto-occipital membrane at the foramen magnum. The posterior longitudinal ligament is connected to the posterior edge of the foramen magnum *via* the membrana tectoria (Fig.1).

The posterior vertebral elements are stabilized by the yellow, interspinous and supraspinous ligaments. The yellow ligament connects the laminae and forms the posterior edge of the spinal canal in the inter-laminar space, and is connected to the skull at the posterior atlanto-occipital membrane. The interspinous ligament serves as an important posterior anchor and passes between the spinous processes, while the supraspinous ligament extends between the tips of the spinous processes.

Both vertebral arteries run through the transverse holes between C6 and C1, although the vertebral artery can enter the cervical spine at other levels such as C3, C4, C5, and C7. In around 89% of cases, the artery passes in a straight line through these transverse holes. Above C2, the artery turns backwards and upwards, crosses the transverse foramen of C1 and continues medially along the upper edge of the atlas in a groove to form a loop towards the dura mater of the foramen magnum (Fig. 4). The vertebral artery is surrounded by a venous plexus which is particularly prominent between C2 and its intracranial segment [145].

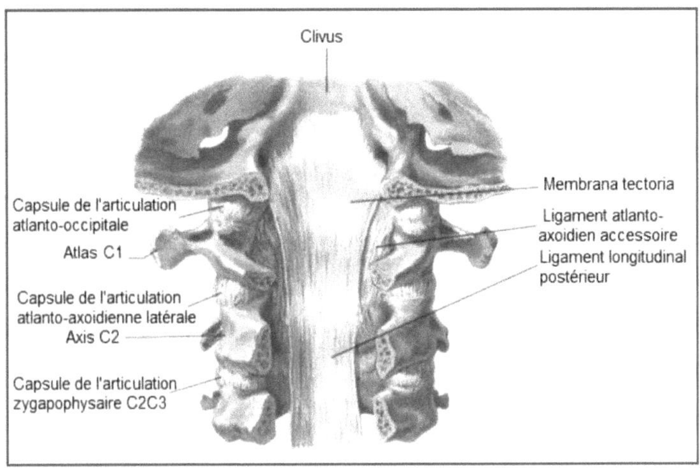

Fig. 1: Posterior view of the occipitovertebral junction after resection of the posterior arches and dural sheath. [92].

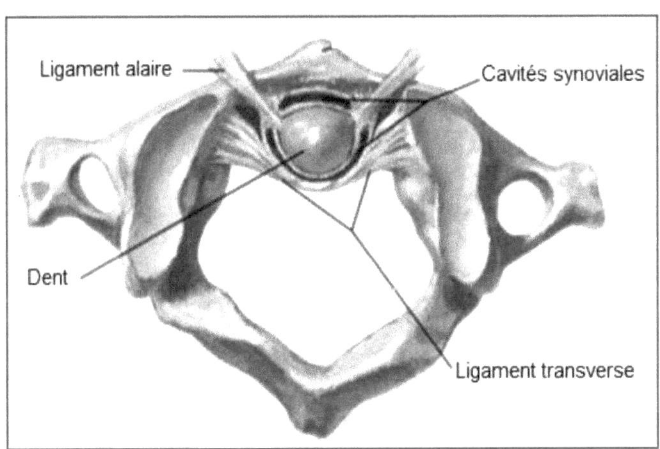

Fig. 2: Superior view of the medial atlantoaxial joint. [92].

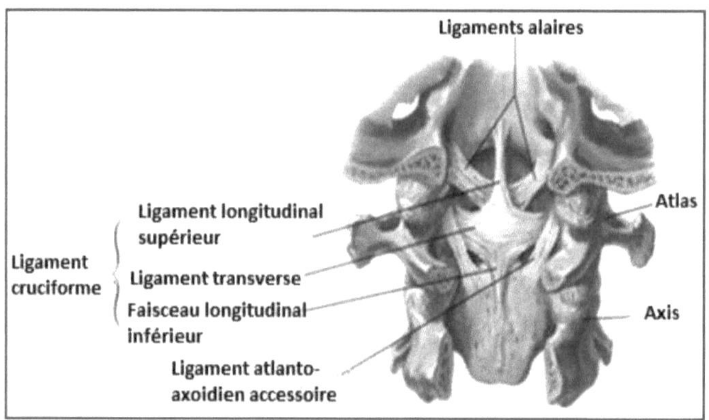

Fig. 3: Posterior view of the deep ligaments exposed after removal of the membrana tectoria. [92].

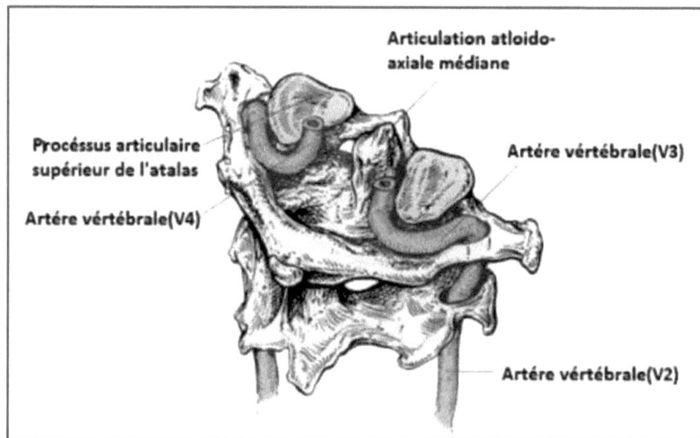

Fig. 4: The vertebral artery. [92].

1.2. Thoracic spine

The 12 thoracic vertebrae are rectangular in shape, with flat upper and lower surfaces. The conjugation holes are almost lateral. The height of the vertebral bodies increases progressively from top to bottom. The intervertebral discs appear flatter than their cervical and lumbar counterparts. The pedicle extends from the upper half of the vertebral body. The semicircular shape of the blades makes the neural canal almost circular, with a constant diameter along the thoracic spine. As this part of the spine is in slight kyphosis, on MRI the dural sac and spinal cord appear slightly displaced forward into the upper thoracic canal (Fig. 5). The major feature of the thoracic spine is the existence of the costovertebral joint(Fig.6).

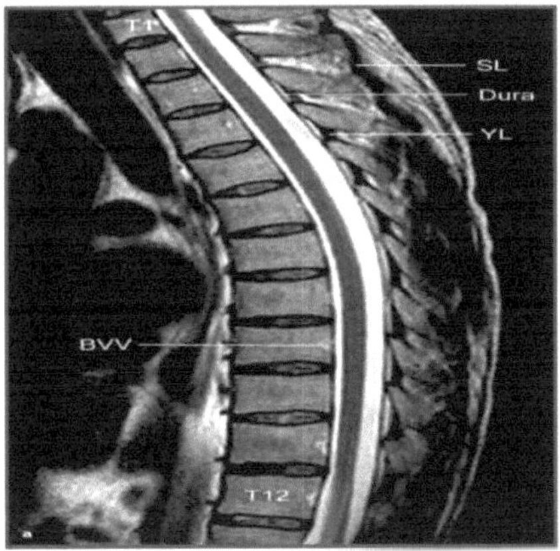

Fig. 5: T2 MRI: Median sagittal section of the thoracic spine.

[**BVV**: Vertebrobasilar vein. **Dura**: dura mater. **SL**: supraspinous ligament. **YL**: Yellow ligament]. [185].

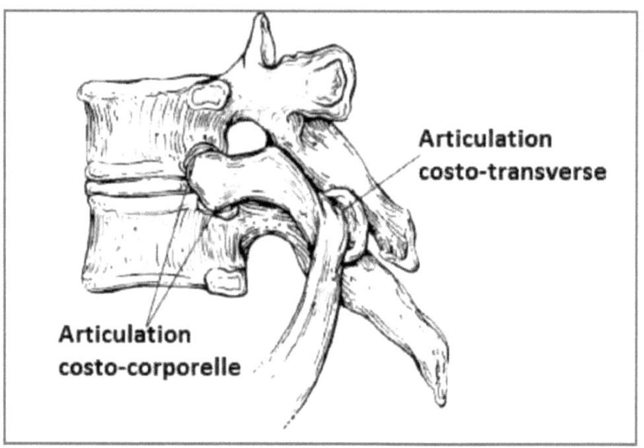

Fig. 6: Lateral view of a costo-vertebral joint. [92].

The external venous plexuses around the vertebral bodies are of particular importance in the thoracic and lumbar region. Changes in intra-thoracic and intra-abdominal pressures are transmitted to the peridural venous plexuses via anastomosis and affect thoracic and lumbar cerebrospinal fluid (CSF) pressure; in addition, there are interconnections between these plexuses and the external azygos venous system.

This connection provides a parallel drainage system that bypasses the superior and inferior vena cava, hence the importance of clearing the abdomen in the ventral position.

1.2. Lumbar spine and sacrum

As with the thoracic vertebrae, the five lumbar vertebrae are made up of rectangular vertebral bodies with flat upper and lower surfaces. The pedicles are oriented posterolaterally. The conjugation holes emerge almost laterally. The posterior edge of each hole is formed by the articular processes. These processes are of constant length and bear the facet joints. The lumbar blades form an oval canal at the top, becoming more triangular at the bottom. The sacrum is composed of four or five fused vertebrae, forming a triangle that articulates laterally with the iliac bone.

1.3. Biomechanics

The line of gravity of the straight human body lies in front of the spine, which is designed in two columns:

➢ The anterior column, made up of the intervertebral bodies and discs, absorbs around 80% of the axial load and supports the distraction forces.

➢ The posterior column, made up of the laminae and articular joints which function as an articular chain controlled by ligaments and muscles, bears the remaining 20% of the axial load as well as the compressive forces, ensuring a balance between the two columns.

Movement of the spine is made possible by deformations of the intervertebral discs and facet joints. Ligaments limit movement.

Stability of the spine requires the integrity of the anterior and posterior elements, so IMT surgery, which requires extensive laminectomies, risks causing deformity and/or instability, particularly in children.

The meninges of the spinal cord differ relatively from those of the encephalon in having a thick pie-mother connected to the medial dural surface by the serrated ligaments, an intermediate leptomeningeal layer and a fatty extradural space (Figs. 7 and 8).

1.4. The dura mater

The dura mater, composed of collagen and elastic fibers, is approximately 0.8 mm thick. It forms a dural sac or dural sheath that encloses the spinal cord, the spinal roots of the spinal nerves, the terminal filum and the ponytail.

The dura mater is separated from the vertebrae by a real extradural space, which is narrower at the front and filled with fat, venous plexuses draining the medulla, and sensory nerves at the front, including Lushka's sinuvertebral nerve, which innervates the ventral part of the dura mater.

If the dura mater has no connection with the dorsal osteo-ligamentary plane, it adheres ventrally to the vertebral ligament via fibrous flanges and to the periosteum in the foramen.

Dural vascularization is ensured by radicular, radiculomedullary and radiculopial arteries [162].

1.5. The arachnoid

The arachnoid is the outer wall of the subarachnoid space, watertight and closely attached to the dura mater. It emits extensions that attach it to the pial surface of the medulla and to the deep surface of the dura, from which it is nevertheless easily detached [185]. Laterally, piebrae and arachnoid are exhausted at the point of contact between nerve and dura mater, which extends into the epinode [159]. In the subarachnoid space, there are several partitions, mainly posterior and to a lesser extent anterior. These partitions are derived from an intermediate fenestrated leptomeningeal membrane, which is attached to the inner surface of the arachnoid and holds nerve roots and blood vessels against the surface of the spinal cord [184].

1.6. The serrated ligament

The serrated ligament, thicker rostrally, is a transverse plate of fibers of a medial pial and lateral dural nature, according to Nauta et al [184]. It transversely binds the two lateral marrow edges to the dural sac like guy wires. The medial edge of each ligament is tighter than the lateral edge, and adheres to the cord opposite the boundary separating the dorsolateral cord from the ventrolateral cord. The outer edge of each ligament forms a succession of arches formed by thick, tooth-like extensions, the apex of which is attached to the dura mater between the overlying and underlying root sheaths. In the cervical region, the ligament lies in front of the accessory nerve.

The cervical teeth are horizontal, while the thoracic teeth are vertical. The first tooth has an ascending direction, surmounting the dural relief of the vertebral artery and attaching immediately above and behind its dural penetration and below and behind the orifice of the XIIème cranial nerve on the margin of the foramen magnum.

The most caudal tooth is thin and filiform, and is inserted above the emergence of the first lumbar nerve. Its medial edge extends into the terminal filum.

When there is one arch per spinal nerve, 21 teeth are counted, but there may be one arch for two nerves and vice versa. The number of teeth thus varies from 18 to 22 for Rabieshang et al [205].

2.4. The mother magpie

The piebrae is made up of loose connective tissue, forming a complex support system that lines the spinal cord [144]. The pietis is not permeable to water and forms a barrier between the subarachnoid space and the perivascular spaces of the medulla [185]. Several observations consider the extracellular space and the subarachnoid space as two compartments of the same liquid space, which allows free circulation between them [211].

This exchange depends on arterial and venous blood flow, and takes place along the DREZ (dorsal root entry zone), where Cloyd et al [43] have demonstrated the existence of fenestrations in the pie-mother.

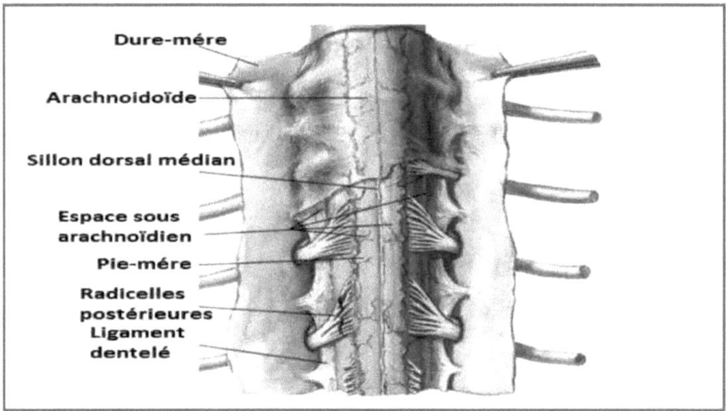

Fig. 7: Posterior view of the thoracic medulla. After opening the dura mater, the meninges are visible with the serrated ligament. [184 bis.]

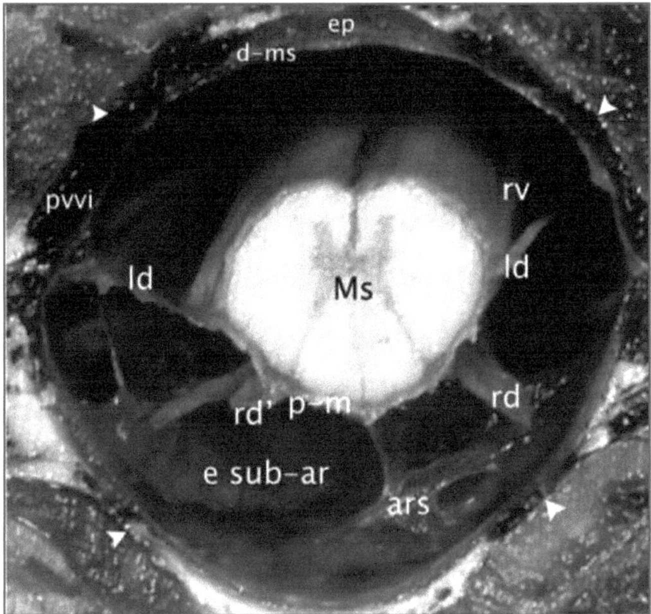

Fig. 8: Axial section of the spinal cord in the spinal canal. **ars**: spinal arachnoid (pressed against the inner surface of the dura mater); **d-ms**: spinal dura mater (constituting the "dural cylindrical sheath"); **ep**: epidural space; **e sub-ar**: sub-arachnoid space (cerebrospinal fluid circulates in this space); **ld**: serrated ligament; **Ms**: spinal cord; **p-m**: perispinous mother lobe (extending laterally through the right and left serrated ligaments); **pvvi**: internal vertebral venous plexus (in epidural space); **rd rd'**: dorsal spinal roots; **rv**: ventral spinal root; **white arrowheads**: mark the perimeter of the vertebral canal. [254].

3. THE SPINAL CORD

The spinal cord is a long, cylindrical cord, flattened from front to back, contained in the vertebral canal. It begins above the emergence of the first cervical root at the occipital foramen (middle of the posterior arch of the atlas) and ends between the 1ere and 2eme lumbar vertebrae (L1L2 disc) (Fig. 7). On average, it measures 1 cm in diameter, 30 grams in weight and 45 cm in length (45.9 cm in men and 41.5 cm in women) [145].

The spinal cord has 4 faces (Fig. 10): ventral, dorsal and two lateral.

• The ventral face is crossed on the median line by the ventral median fissure (or scissure), 2 to 3 mm deep, whose lips can be spread as far as the anterior white commissure. This fissure separates the ventral face into two symmetrical ventral cords, 2 to 3 mm wide, and is limited by two ventro-lateral grooves from which the ventral roots emerge.

• The dorsal side features the median dorsal septum (or groove) on the midline, and dorso-lateral grooves laterally, from which the dorsal roots emerge.

• The lateral faces between the ventro-lateral and dorso-lateral sulci.

The spinal cord also has 2 bulges that correspond to a greater density of neurons destined for the limbs:

■ Cervical bulge: between C4 and C7, more pronounced at C5 C6 corresponds to the medullary segments from C5 to T1, from which the nerves for the upper limbs originate.

■ Lumbar bulge: extends from T9 to T12, corresponds to the medullary segments from T10 to L5, from which the nerves for the lower limbs originate, and surmounts the *terminal cone,* which ends like the tip of a blunt at the L1L2 disc.

Between the two bulges lies the *thoracic medulla,* which contains fewer neurons and is therefore smaller in diameter.

The *terminal filum, an* atrophied remnant of the caudal segment of the medulla, extends from the medullary cone to the dorsal surface of the coccyx. It is formed by condensation of pie-mother and leaves the dural sac at the level of the second sacral vertebra, forming the coccygeal ligament which continues to the dorsal surface of the coccyx.

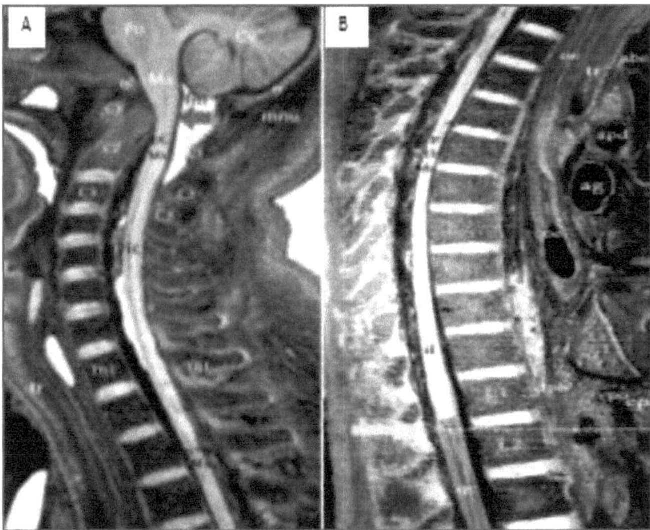

Fig. 9: Median sagittal section of the spinal cord. **C1**: atlas; **C2**: axis; **C3**: 3eme cervical vertebra, **Cv**: cerebellum; **fm**: foramen magnum; **ic**: cervical intumescence (vertebral levels: C3 to Th1).**Ma**: elongated medulla; **pCMs**: cervical part of the spinal cord (vertebral levels: C1 and C2); **Po**: bridge; **pTh**: thoracic part of the medulla (vertebral levels: Th2 to Th9); **Th2**: 2ème thoracic vertebra; **red arrows**: mark the cranial end of the medulla (level corresponding to a narrowing: the isthmus of the encephalon"). **Com**: medullary cone; **il**: lumbar intumescence; **L1**: 1ère lumbar vertebra; **L2**: 2ème lumbar vertebra; **pThMs**: thoracic part of the spinal cord; **qc**: ponytail; **yellow arrow** marking the level of the caudal end of the spinal cord (upper edge of L2). [254].

3.2. Internal configuration

The spinal cord is made up of deep *gray matter* and peripheral *white matter*. In the center is the ependymal duct.

3.2.1. Gray matter

The gray matter is divided into dorsal and ventral horns. It is also divided according to Cytoarchitectonic criteria into 10 dorso-ventral zones known as Rexed layers (Fig. 10).

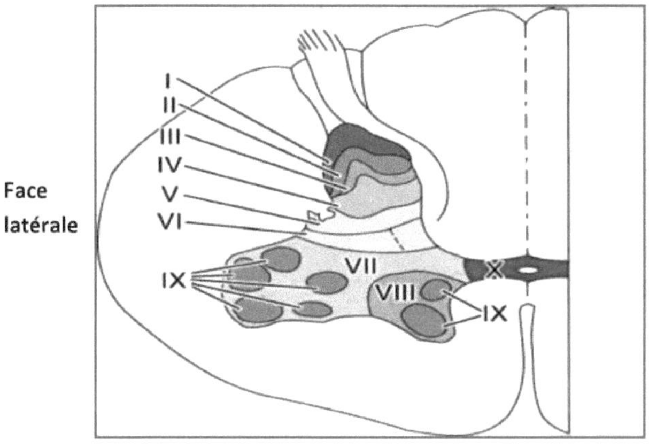

Fig. 10: Gray matter at C6 organized into Rexed layers. [186].

• Dorsal horns: (layers I to VI) receive incoming afferent nerve fibres from dorsal roots.

• Ventral horns: (layers VII-VIII to X) contain, among other things, motor neurons which project via ventral roots to skeletal muscles. Rexed layer IX corresponds to striated muscle motor neurons.

• The intermediolateral horns: (layer VII) located on the thoracic and upper lumbar segments contain the cell bodies of pre-ganglionic sympathetic neurons. At sacral level (S2-S4), they contain pre-ganglionic parasympathetic neurons.

3.2.2. White matter

The white matter is organized into cords, which contain the long tracts (descending and ascending) (Fig. 11) :

• Ventral cords: between the ventral median scissure and the ventro-lateral sulcus.

• The lateral cords: between the ventro-lateral sulci and the dorso-lateral sulci.

• The dorsal cords: between the dorso-lateral sulci and the dorsal median sulcus.

3.2.2.1. Descending or motor pathways

The descending or motor pathways are essentially composed of pyramidal or cortico-spinal fascicles.

➢ The cross-pyramidal bundle is the most important, occupying the posterior region of the lateral cord, with somatotopic fibers (medial fibers for cervical use, lateral fibers for sacral use).

At the level of each metamerion, the fibers leave the pyramidal tract and enter the ventral horn medioventrally at the level of lamina VII, where they articulate with the second motor neurons forming the ventral root.

➢ The direct pyramidal bundle (less than 20% of pyramidal fibers), which runs in the ventral cord, flush with the ventral median fissure, is destined for the cervical muscles and is bilaterally distributed.

➢ The extrapyramidal bundles originating from the supra-segmental centers of the brain stem are arranged in two contingents:

• The anteromedial (vestibulospinal, medial reticulospinal, olivospinal, tectospinal and interstitial spinal bundles), whose fibers in the ventral cord terminate bilaterally in the ventral horn (lamina VII), exert a facilitating action on postural tone (extensor and axial antigravitational muscles).

- The other, posterolateral (rubro-spinal, retuculo-spinal bundle of bulbar origin), whose fibers also terminate homo- or contralaterally in lamina VII of the ventral horn, exerts a facilitating action on the distal flexors.

3.2.2.2. Ascending or sensory pathways

In the ascending or sensory pathways, we distinguish three types of fascicles:

➢ Goll (or gracile) and Burdach (or cuneiform) fascicles, located together in the dorsal cord, directly and ipsilaterally convey conscious proprioceptive information (joint movement and position) and discriminatory touch to the Goll and Burdach nuclei of the inferior bulb.

➢ Spino-thalamic bundle, located in the ventro-lateral cord, transports information related to algic and thermal sensations, as well as to non-discriminatory touch and pressure, to the thalamus, after a segmental relay.

➢ Dorsal (or Flechsig's bundle) and ventral (or Gowers' bundle) spino-cerebellar fascicles, located near the dorso-lateral and ventro-lateral surfaces respectively, transport information from muscle spindles, Golgi tendon organs and tactile receptors to the cerebellum for posture control and movement coordination.

3.2.3. The central or ependymal duct

The central canal runs the full height of the medulla and is a vestige of the embryonic neural canal, which rarely remains in adults (Fig.11).

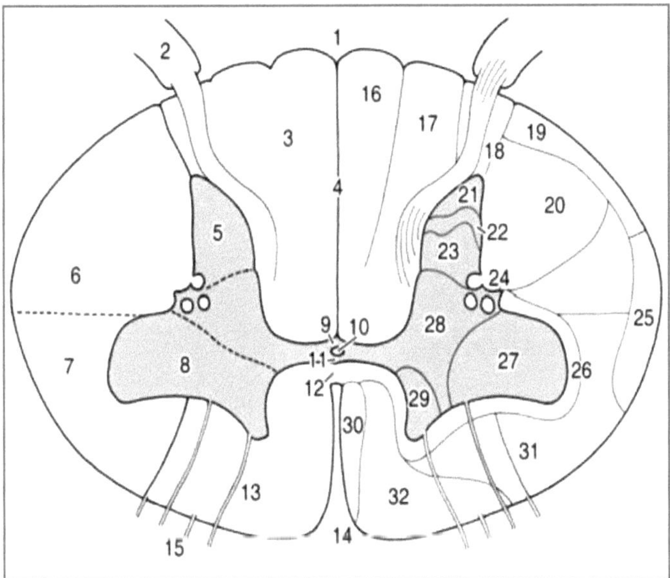

Fig. 11: Axial section of medulla: 1. posterior median groove, 2. dorsal root, 3. posterior cord, 4. posterior median groove, 5. dorsal horn, 6. posterolateral cord, 7. anterolateral cord, 8. anterior horn, 9. Posterior gray commissure, 10. central canal, 11. anterior gray commissure, 12. ventral commissure (white), 13. anterior cord, 14. anterior median groove, 15. anterior root, 16. gracile bundle, 17. wedge-shaped bundle, 18. Dorsolateral bundle, 19. Dorsal spinal-cerebellar bundle, 20. Lateral pyramidal bundle (crossed), 21. Dorsal horn (lamina I), 22. Dorsal horn (lamina II and III), 23. Dorsal horn (lamina IV), 24. Intermediate zone (processus reticularis), 25. Ventral spinal-cerebellar fascicle, 26. proper fascicle, 27. lateral motor spine (lamina IX), 28. intermediate zone (lamina V-VIII), 29. medial motor spine (lamina IX), 30. direct pyramidal fascicle, 31. anterolateral fascicle, 32.

Mediolateral bundle. [186].

3.3. Vascularization

Medullary vascularization is one of the most complex in the body, due to the large number of arteries that contribute to it.

3.3.1. Arterial supply

Arterial supply is provided by the radiculo-medullary arteries, the number and origin of which depend on each territory (Fig.12).

The entire medullary cord is supplied by only 6 to 8 anterior medullary-radicular arteries and around twenty posterior medullary-radicular arteries. This supply is organized into 3 different vascular territories [252].

3.3.1.1. The cervical region

The cervical territory is supplied at two levels.

➢ High cervical (C0 to C3): there are no radiculo-medullary arteries, and the supply is provided by 2 spinal arteries arising from the termination of each vertebral artery, as are the two posterior spinal arteries.

➢ Middle and low cervical (C4 to T3): there are usually two main anterior medullary-radicular arteries, one arising from the vertebral artery opposite the C5C6 or C4C5 conjugation foramen, and the other, known as the cervical bulge artery, arising from the deep cervical artery and entering the canal via the C7T1 conjugation foramen.

Three to four posterior medullary-radicular arteries, derived from the vertebral artery, supply the posterior spinal tracts.

3.3.1.2. The intermediate or middle thoracic territory (T3-T9)

A single anterior medullary-radicular artery usually arises from the dorsospinal branch of the T4 or T5 intercostal artery, usually at

artery. This artery is often small, with little or no possibility of supplementation. Four to nine posterior medullary arteries feed this segment.

3.3.1.3. The lower or thoraco-lumbar territory (T10-L1)

The anterior spinal axis most often receives a single, voluminous afference, the Adamkiewiez artery or lumbar bulge artery (Fig. 10). Its origin lies on the left side in 70% of cases, and between T9 and L2 in 80% of cases. When the origin of the Adamkiewiz is low, there is a radiculo-medullary artery on the $8^{éme}$, $9^{éme}$ or $10^{éme}$ thoracic root, and conversely when its origin is high, an additional radiculo-medullary artery follows the last lumbar or sacral roots, arising from a lateral lumbar or sacral artery [63].

Four to eight posterior medullary-radicular arteries arise from the intercostal and lumbar arteries, vascularizing the posterior spinal axes. Two of these correspond to the posterior spinal arteries of the cone, usually arising between T12 and L3, and anastomosing at the end of the cone with the terminus of the Adamkiewiz artery, forming the anastomotic loop of the cone or anastomotic basket of the cone.

3.3.2. The perimedullary and intramedullary network

The longitidunal *perimedullary network,* together with the *transverse network,* forms a grid that gives rise to the intramedullary arteries.

3.3.2.1. Perimedullary arteries

They are organized into three distinct longitudinal pathways (the medial anterior spinal axis and the two posterolateral streams) (Fig. 12) and horizontal pathways.

• Anterior spinal artery: the anterior spinal artery arises from the union of two descending branches of the vertebral arteries, generally at the level of the foramen magnum, more rarely at cervical level. It is possible to observe a double anterior spinal artery over almost the entire spinal cord, but more often than not, these splits are only observed over a few centimetres.

The anterior spinal artery runs in the anterior median scissure, and its diameter is larger at the lumbosacral level than at the dorsal level; but variations are possible at different levels. The diameter of the anterior spinal artery is larger after junction with an arterial inflow.

Blood flow in the anterior spinal artery is generally downward from cervical to lumbosacral level.

• Posterior spinal arteries: the two posterior spinal arteries arise either directly from the vertebral artery or from the posteroinferior cerebellar arteries. They are usually two tortuous arteries descending laterally towards the DREZ, in the posterolateral part of the medulla (Fig. 14).

Blood flow in the posterior spinal arteries is descending at cervical and dorsal level, and ascending at lumbosacral level.

- Horizontal pathways: the horizontal pathways, also known as the "perimedullary coronary anastomotic network", unite the preceding longitudinal pathways to form a perimedullary crown from which medullary perforating branches emerge (Fig. 13).

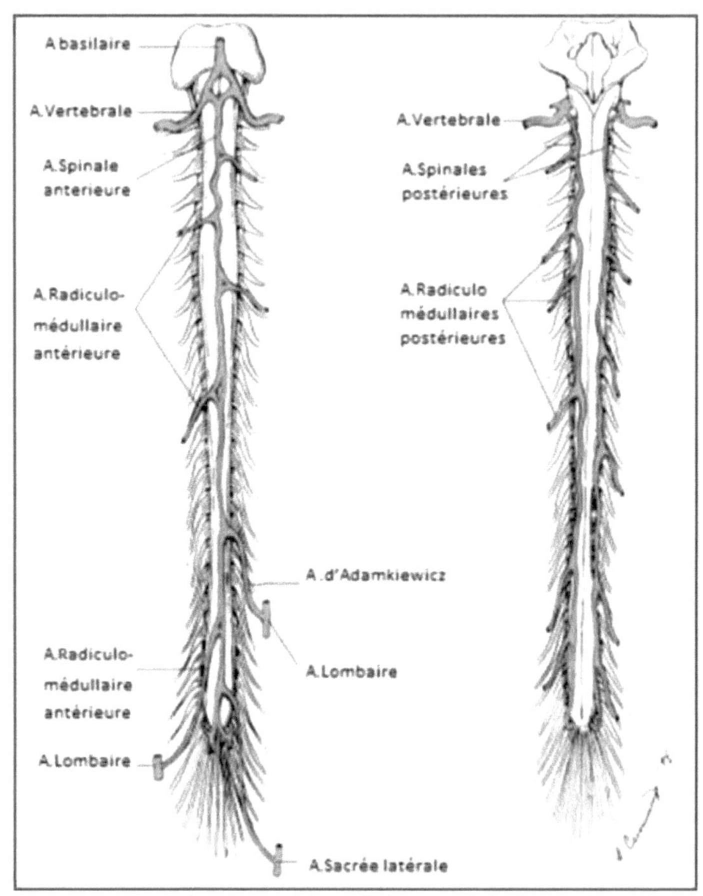

Fig. 12: Arterial supply (A: artery). [92].

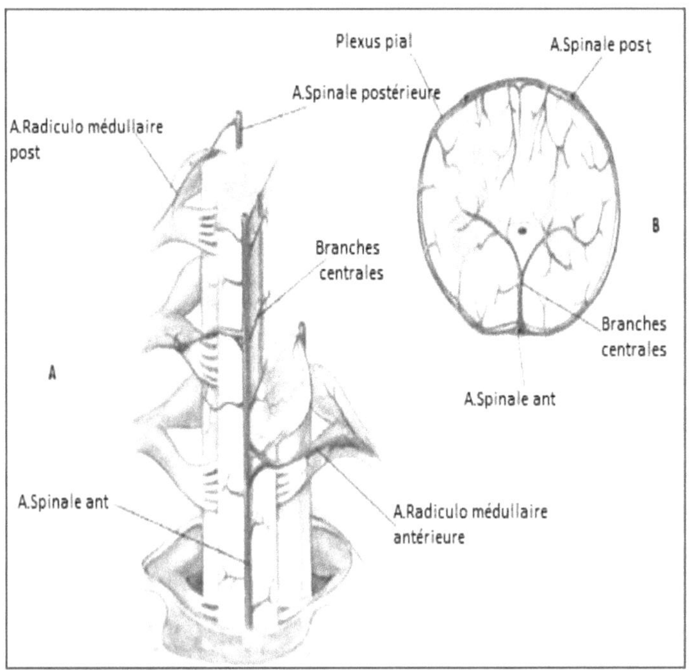

Fig. 13: Organization of the arterial vascularization of the medulla. **A**: Root arteries feeding the spinal arteries, which give rise to the central branches. **B**: Vascular territories of the anterior and posterior spinal arteries. [92].

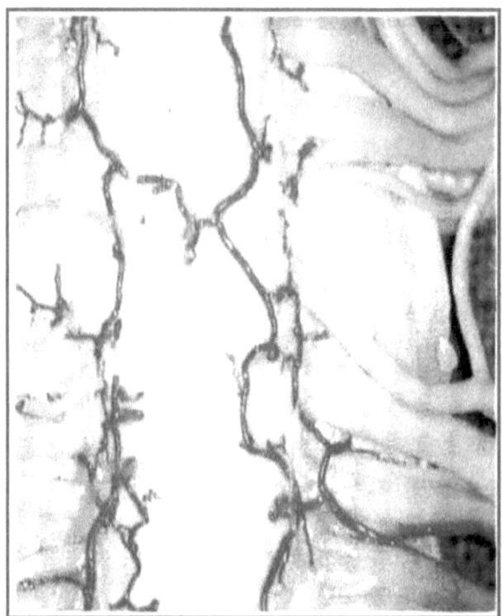

Fig. 14: Posterior view of the thoracic medulla. The two posterior spinal arteries are visible. [79].

3.3.2.2. The intramedullary arterial network

The intramedullary arterial network is made up of multiple peripheral perforating and central or sulco-commissural branches:

• Multiple peripheral perforating branches originating from the pial network penetrate the peripheral white matter of the anterolateral and posterior cords.

• Central or sulco-commissural branches (180 to 200 in total) arise from the anterior spinal axis and enter horizontally into the anterior medial sulcus, dividing into multiple branches that vascularize the anterior cords and gray matter, with the exception of the posterior part of the posterior horns.

The anterior spinal pathway vascularizes a central territory irrigated by the sulco-commissural arteries, representing 80% of spinal cord vascularization and including virtually all the white matter of the anterolateral cords, including the pyramidal bundle.

Whereas the peripheral territory irrigated by the pial network includes virtually all the white matter of the posterior cords and the gray matter of the head of the posterior horn, there are no anastomoses in the medulla, whose penetrating vessels are essentially terminal.

3.3.3. Venous efferences

Intramedullary and perimedullary veins and pure root veins join the longitudinal spinal veins on the ventral and dorsal surface of the medulla, from which blood leaves the intradural sector via the medullary-radicular veins to join the epidural veins.

The straight anterior median spinal vein runs in the anterior median groove and receives collaterals from the anterior veins of the ponytail, lumbar and dorsal roots.

The posterior spinal vein (Fig. 15) runs in the posterior and lateral sulci of the medulla. It is formed at the base by the union of all the veins of the ponytail roots and the terminal filum. At all levels, it receives veins from the roots, the venules of the posterior surface of the medulla and the conus. It is single and median at the lumbar and cervical levels, but two or even three dorsal longitudinal veins are observed at the thoracic level.

The anterior and posterior medullo-radicular veins drain the anterior and posterior spinal veins into the extradural spaces.

As they pass through the dura mater, these veins take on a chicane shape, narrowing in caliber and altering in morphology to form an anti-reflux device. Opposite the holes of conjugation, they drain into the spinal epidural plexuses:

- **At** cervical level, into the superior vena cava *via* the deep cervical vertebral veins and posterior jugular veins.

In the thoracic region, via intercostal veins into the great azygos vein on the right, and into the superior and inferior hemi-azygos veins on the left.

- At lumbar level, in ascending lumbar veins.

- At the sacral level, in the sacral and hypogastric veins, joining the inferior vena cava.

The anterior and posterior spinal veins also drain directly, upwards into the cranial sinuses and downwards into the vein of the terminal filum.

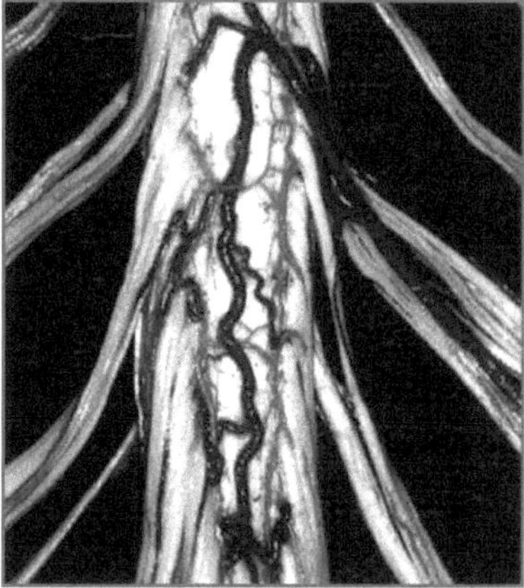

Fig. 15: Posterior view of the thoracic medulla. After opening the dura mater, the posterior median venous axis can be visualized. [79].

4. NERVE ROOTS AND SPINAL NERVES

Sensory fibres with spinal ganglia containing cell bodies enter the spinal cord via the posterior roots in the DREZ, while motor fibres containing motor neuron axons (their cell bodies are located in the medullary grey matter) leave the cord *via* the anterior roots in the DREZ.

at the level of the corresponding ventral surface of the medulla. Anastomoses exist between posterior roots in the subarachnoid space between neighbouring segments in less than 61% of cases. Such anastomoses are much rarer between the fibers of the anterior roots, and have only been identified in around 21% [144]. The posterior and anterior roots traverse the subarachnoid space in a laterocaudal direction and in most cases penetrate the dura mater in separate sheaths (Figs. 7 and 8).

The arachnoid fuses with the anterior and posterior roots several millimeters medial to the spinal ganglion and merges with the root dura mater sleeve [145]. The dorsal root ganglion lies posteriorly in the foramen of conjugation just medial to the junction between the dorsal and ventral roots (Figs. 7 and 8).

Connective tissue, fat and vascular structures surround the spinal nerve in its foramen magnum, with the venous plexus being its most important structure.

There are 31 pairs of spinal nerves emerging from the medulla: there are 8 pairs of cervical nerves (C1 to C8), 12 pairs of thoracic nerves (T1 to T12), 5 pairs of lumbar nerves (L1 to L5), 5 pairs of sacral nerves (S1 to S5) and 1 pair of coccygeal nerves. The first seven pairs of spinal nerves (C1 -C7) exit the vertebral canal above their respective cervical vertebrae, while from C8 onwards they exit below their corresponding vertebrae (this is due to the fact that there are 7 cervical vertebrae for 8 pairs of cervical nerves).

Note that at cervical level, the roots are practically horizontal due to the termination of the spinal cord at the L2 vertebra, while at lumbosacral level, the roots become vertical, forming the cauda equina.

For the vegetative functions of spinal nerves, there are sympatho-afferent and sympatho-efferent fibers [144].

IV. SEMIOLOGY

The clinical picture is characteristic of the state phase and includes a lesion syndrome, a sub-lesion syndrome and a spinal syndrome. The clinical presentation of TIM is variable, however, and can take any form of slow spinal cord compression.

1. EPIDEMIOLOGICAL DATA

IMTs account for 2-4% of primary tumors of the central nervous system, and 30% of intradural intrarachid tumors [206-217]. According to a report by the French Society of Neurosurgery (SFNC) [79], their incidence is estimated at 4 cases per million inhabitants per year, compared with 6.5 cases per million inhabitants per year in the USA [35].

1.1. Age of onset

IMTs occur most frequently in young adults, with an average age ranging from 36 to 43 years, and are rare in children, when they are most often astrocytomas [70-114-183-206-263-265].

1.2. Gender

Fischer [79] found a slight male predominance, while Issaacson [114] reported a discrete female predominance.

2. PATHOPHYSIOLOGY

The pathophysiological mechanisms that generate the symptoms of slow cord compression are specific to each of the 3 syndromes.

2.1. Spinal syndrome

The spinal syndrome is explained by the suffering of the osteo-igamentary apparatus opposite the lesion in relation to a symptomatic segmental deformity (e.g. kyphosis symptomatic of TIM in children).

2.2. Lesion syndrome

The lesion syndrome is metameric and corresponds to irritation or compression of the root opposite the lesion in question.

2.3. Subinjury syndrome

Sublesional syndrome is explained by suffering of the motor and sensory pathways due to mechanical compression of the spinal cords by the lesion and/or circulatory insufficiency. This suffering is expressed throughout the territory below the lesion. The upper limit of the sub-lesional syndrome and the metameric lesional syndrome together clinically designate the level of the lesion, a key clinical element in the orientation of explorations before the advent of MRI.

3. DIAGNOSTIC

The diagnosis of spinal cord compression requires specialist advice from the very first clinical signs, as it requires urgent treatment.

3.1. Clinical diagnosis

The onset of clinical signs is usually gradual, insidious and not very disabling, lasting weeks, months or even years.

The alarm is sometimes given by motor disorders, essentially fatigability when walking, but in the vast majority of cases, the pain can affect all types: radicular, cordonal or spinal.

A positive diagnosis of spinal cord injury must be made as soon as possible, because the quality of the outcome, in terms of both surgical procedure and prognosis, is directly related to the extent of neurological damage at the time of diagnosis and treatment.

3.1.1. Start stage

It is at this early stage that the diagnosis must be made, looking carefully for signs related to the three more or less interrelated syndromes: spinal, lesional and sub-lesional.

3.1.1.1. Spinal syndrome

If spinal pain is segmental and persistent, with nocturnal recrudescence, even in the absence of spontaneous pain, it should be investigated:

- segmental stiffness of the spine.

- localized pain on pressure and percussion of the spinous processes.

- spinal deformity, especially in children.

These signs do not necessarily indicate the bony origin of the compression.

3.1.1.2. Lesion syndrome

The lesion syndrome is highly localizing (essential dermatomes: T1 level corresponds to the upper edge of the sternal manubrium, T4 to the nipple line, T6 to the tip of the xiphoid, T10 to the o mbilic and L1 to the pubis and groin folds) and precedes the sub-lesion syndrome. There are no neurological signs above the lesion level.

Subjective signs

Radicular pain is very typical in that it covers the territory of one or more roots (pain in a limb or chest pain in a belt), has a precise, fixed and constant topography in the same patient, is very sharp in a flash, neuralgic in nature, rebellious and impulsive when coughing or exerting oneself. Paradoxically, they are sometimes accentuated by rest and decubitus, and when nocturnal, they prevent sleep (standing pain). Paresthesias are unpleasant sensations of tingling, prickling or numbness that can be felt in the extremities.

Objective signs

Deficient radicular symptoms go unnoticed in the thoracic region, but are very debilitating in the cervical and lumbar regions. In the same metameric radicular territory as the pain, look for :
- hypoesthesia in radicular bands in the painful territory.
- abolition of a reflex.
- a radicular motor deficit.

3.1.1.3. Subinjury syndrome

Subinjury syndrome is often discreet at this early stage, and usually presents with motor disorders associated with sensory disturbances.

Motor disorders

Motor disorders often present with a number of signs, including :

➤ *Subjective signs:* usually begin in the lower limbs with motor fatigability, difficulty running and then walking, sometimes true painless intermittent claudication, spasmodic stiffness of the lower limbs. Fatigue is followed by functional motor discomfort, then motor deficits in both lower limbs, which progressively set in, with occasional clumsiness of an upper limb.

➤ *Objective signs*: at this stage, the examination reveals a discrete pyramidal syndrome marked by a slight reduction in muscle strength, predominantly in the shortening muscles of the lower limbs. On the other hand, reflex changes are very important, and should be carefully examined for osteotendinous hyperreflexia. Abdominal cutaneous reflexes are diminished or abolished.

Sensory disorders

Like the first, sensory disorders also present themselves with a certain number of signs that we present in succession:

➤ *subjective signs*: bilateral posterior cord pain throughout the sub-lesional territory. These are either sudden attacks of pain (pain in a flash, sensation of electric discharge) or paresthesias of the tingling type, sensation of constriction in a vice, sensation of cold or hot water trickling down, sensation of walking on absorbent cotton.

Sometimes the pain is of the spinothalamic type: sensations of burning or cooking on a permanent painful background in an area of thermo-algesic hypoesthesia.

Barefoot walkers may have difficulty perceiving the ground, causing walking difficulties, especially with eyes closed, and progressing to full-blown sensory ataxia.

> *Objective signs*: sensory deficits in all modes of sensibility, posterior cord (discriminative sensitivity) and spinothalamic (thermo-algesic sensitivity).

Posterior cord syndrome caused by damage to the lemniscal pathway includes disorders of position and movement involving proprioceptive afferents (so-called deep sensitivity disorders), reduction or loss of sense of segmental attitudes, sensory ataxia (Romberg's sign), unstable ataxic hand (outstretched hand test, eyes closed), failure of blind grasping (finger on nose, heel on knee), reduction or abolition of vibratory sense (pallesthesia) and disorders of sensory perception, eyes closed), blind prehension failure (finger on nose, heel on knee), decreased or abolished vibratory sense (pallesthesia) and disorders of superficial epicritic fine discriminative sensitivity, disorders of spatial discrimination, topographical accuracy (topoesthesia) and weight assessment (baresthesia). These disorders of sensitive discrimination may be responsible for astereognosia or loss of graphesthesia.

Spinothalamic syndrome caused by damage to the extra-lemniscal pathway involves altered thermo-algesic sensitivity, i.e. sensitivity to pain, heat and cold, and protopathic tactile sensitivity.

The upper limit of disorders is usually clear-cut and corresponds to the level of the lesion syndrome.

In addition, sexual disorders (frigidity, impotence) and vesicosphincter disorders (urgent micturition followed by retention and overflow micturition, constipation or incontinence) can be part of the above picture.

3.1.2. Advanced stage

The three syndromes are grouped and progressively accentuated, and it is the intensity of the sub-injury syndrome that determines the severity of the picture.

3.1.2.1. Motor disorders

Decreased muscle strength is assessed globally using the Barré maneuver for the upper limbs and the Mingazzini and Barré maneuver for the lower limbs; segmental assessment may be required in some cases. A frank muscular deficit should therefore be sought by testing muscle strength, which is rated from 0 to 5 :

0 = No contraction.

1 = Visible contraction without movement.

2 = Contraction allowing movement in the absence of gravity.

3 = Contraction allowing movement against gravity.

4 = Contraction allowing movement against resistance.

5 = Normal muscle strength.

So we can find :

Tetra/Paraparesis or even spastic tetra/paraplegia, where walking becomes difficult or impossible.

Osteotendinous reflexes are sharp, diffuse and polykinetic. There is clonus of the patella, inexhaustible trepidation of the foot and bilateral Babinski's sign.

Pyramidal hypertonicity is permanent, exaggerated by voluntary movements and predominantly in the extensors. Defense reflexes are easily triggered.

3.1.2.2. Sensory disorders

Sensory disturbances involve all modes of sensitivity, resulting in hypoesthesia or even anesthesia, the upper limit of which approaches the lesion level as it progresses.

3.1.2.3. Sphincter and trophic disorders

Major sphincter disorders, non-use amyotrophy, pressure sores, thromboembolism and infections are complications that occur at a stage of myelomalacia with complete flaccid tetra/paraplegia.

3.2. Clinical forms

We distinguish between clinical forms based on the location of the lesion, as well as forms in children and forms with a sudden onset.

3.2.1. In height

Since semiology depends on the location of the lesion in height, we need to make a clinical distinction between cervical, dorsal, lumbar and terminal cone forms.

 ➤ *The cervical cord*, which manifests itself as tetraparesis and then spastic tetraplegia, with further topographical variations:

- The bulbous-medullary junction is enriched by involvement of the last four cranial nerves.

- Level C4 involves paralysis of the diaphragm due to phrenic damage, causing respiratory distress, and level C2 involves neuralgia of Arnold's great nerve.

- The cervico-dorsal junction may involve only partial involvement of the upper limbs. T1 involvement is responsible for Claude-Bernard-Horner syndrome.

▷ *As for the dorsal medulla,* its damage is revealed by paraparesis and then spastic paraplegia, with the only variations being height references. The radicular pain associated with dorsal compression is very typical in the girdle or hemi-girdle. The level of the radicular pain and the upper limit of the sub-lesional sensory deficit together define the level of the lesion. Sometimes, the pain associated with the lesion syndrome may suggest a visceral disorder.

> *Lumbar spinal cord* and *conus medullaris,* including the lumbar bulge extending from T10 to L2. Symptoms include flaccid paralysis of the lower limbs (as in ponytail syndrome) and pyramidal irritation syndrome with bilateral Babinski sign and, above all, spastic neuro-bladder.

3.2.2. In width

Depending on the location of the lesion in relation to the width of the different cords and the center of the spinal cord, we distinguish between different neurological pictures, which we present in turn as follows:

- Lateral compression of the spinal cord is responsible for Brown-Séquard syndrome, which combines pyramidal syndrome and posterior cord syndrome on the side with spinothalamic deficit on the opposite side.

- Posterior compression of the spinal cord is responsible for a posterior cord syndrome combining pain, Lhermitte's sign (shooting pain along the back, triggered by flexion of the cervical spine) and posterior cord sensory deficit.

- Anterior cord compression is responsible for an early pyramidal syndrome and spinothalamic deficit.

- Centromedullary compression is responsible for a suspended-band thermo-algesic anesthesia, known as "syringomyelic-type dissociation".

3.2.3. Acute paintings

This is an extreme emergency, with major spinal cord damage occurring very rapidly, sometimes preceded by spinal pain. When faced with this situation, it is essential to look for TIM before talking about myelitis or myelomalacia.

3.2.4. Childhood IMD

The clinical picture differs little from that of adults, but it is always more difficult to identify spinal or radicular pain. In small children, on the other hand, spinal deformities such as scoliosis, kyphosis or stilted head carriage can be observed very early on [23].

Occasionally, IMT may present as intracranial hypertension with papilledema or hydrocephalus secondary to circulatory blockage of the CSF. Some cases present with abdominal pain, necessitating extensive gastrointestinal investigations before arriving at a diagnosis of IMT [II7].

Standard radiographs are still very useful, as IMT at this age often results in bone abnormalities [266].

3.3. Functional assessment

Several scores are used for functional assessment of patients with IMD, the most widely used in the literature being the McCormick score.

Other publications use the Frankel or Karnowsky classifications [83-133-206].

Table I: McCormick's modified functional classification [165].

GRADE	DESCRIPTION
I	- No deficit, more or less minimal dysesthesia. - Normal operation.
II	- Minimal deficiency, not affecting function. - Normal operation.
III	- Moderate sensory or motor deficit affecting function. - Moderate walking difficulty. - Severe pain degrading quality of life. - Maintaining independence.
IV	- More severe deficiency. - Walking with canes and/or significant loss of upper limb function. - Need for occasional help.
V	- Severe deficit with impossible walking. - Loss of autonomy.

3.4. Differential diagnosis

When faced with a medullary symptomatology, diagnostic problems no longer arise in the same way as before the MRI era, when other etiologies could be overlooked:

- Paraplegia of central origin due to compression of the two paracentral lobules by certain brain scythe meningiomas when no encephalic symptoms attract attention.

- In pure myelitis (transverse myelitis), the onset of neurological signs is variable: acute onset in less than 24 hours is not uncommon, and the deficit reaches its peak between 1 and 10 days in 50% of subjects.

A viral infection in the days or weeks preceding the onset of myelitis is found in a third of cases.

Spinal cord MRI is normal in 40-50% of cases. The most frequent abnormality is the presence of one or more hypersignals on T2-weighted sequences. On T1-weighted sequences, there may be an increase in marrow volume or a hypo signal. Lesions may enhance after gadolinium injection. At a distance, severe atrophy may be observed. Independently of treatment of the cause, where present, treatment in the acute phase is based on corticosteroids.

- Biermer's anemia, which combines neurological disorders with digestive manifestations, is confirmed by myelograms showing megaloblastic anemia and by a drop in serum vitamin B12 levels. Vitamin B12 treatment improves clinical signs.

- Today, multiple sclerosis in the spinal cord is confirmed much more on the basis of spinal cord and encephalic MRI than on the basis of the three potentials and/or biological criteria. Imaging shows multiple disseminated plaques, likely to fade spontaneously or under the influence of corticosteroid therapy.

- Amyotrophic lateral sclerosis is a neuromuscular disorder, confirmed by the EnMG study, which shows peripheral neurogenic muscle damage.

3.5. Further tests

The management of IMT has undergone real change, thanks to the development of and access to MRI. In fact, MRI is the only complementary examination that has become indispensable for the diagnosis and follow-up of IMT. Other examinations (X-rays, CT scans, evoked potentials, arteriography) are still widely used.

3.5.1. Imaging

The radiological tests that can be requested as part of an investigation into spinal cord disease are standard X-rays, CT scans, myelography, spinal arteriography and MRI. The latter has undoubtedly revolutionized diagnostic methods, unless contraindicated, in which case CT scans and/or myelography take over.

3.5.1.1. Standard X-rays

Standard X-rays are still performed to analyze the morphology and statics of the spine, particularly of the affected segment, and to facilitate anatomical location of the correct lesion level pre- or intraoperatively. In rare cases of slowly progressing TIM, we may observe erosion of a pedicle, or scalopping of the posterior wall, or widening of the spinal canal. Static disorders such as straightness of the cervical spine with disappearance of physiological lordosis may be the telltale sign of IMT, particularly in children [154].

If recurrence is to be investigated, dynamic X-rays are useful for ruling out iatrogenic instability, which should be taken into consideration.

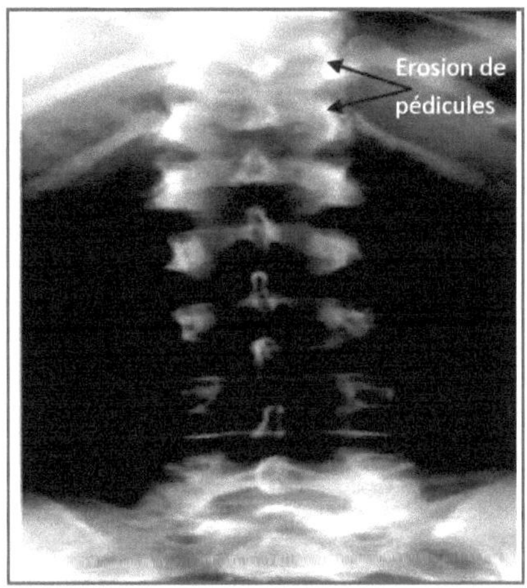

Fig. 16: Frontal dorsolumbar spine radiograph showing pedicle erosion. [133].

3.5.1.2. Myelography, CT and myeloscanner

Myelography, CT scan and myeloscanner are indicated when MRI is contraindicated and/or unavailable. They are capable of demonstrating a large cord without etiological arguments. Myelography is the first-line examination when the level of injury is uncertain, and in the absence of MRI. It pinpoints the site of compression. Stopping of the progression of the contrast medium is sometimes suggestive of the etiology: stop in the shape of a flute-beak or combed appearance in the case of extradural compression, stop in the shape of a dome or cup in the case of a meningioma or neuroma. IMTs are revealed by a fusiform image. Once the level has been determined, a myeloscan centered on the lesion site may show a cystic component, hypodensity of a large lipoma, calcification or an area of hyperdensity within the medulla after intravenous injection of contrast medium.

3.5.1.2. MRI

MRI is the examination of choice, thanks to its high contrast resolution and multiplanar study, and is the first-line examination for all cases of spinal cord compression. The entire spine and cord are scanned in sagittal, axial and sometimes coronal sequences to obtain an optimal lesion assessment [26].

- *T 1 sequences*: anatomical sequence providing an excellent morphological image of the medulla, spine and peri-spinal soft tissues. It can show a large spinal cord on one or more levels, as well as the level of the tumor, which is located in relation to the spine.

- *T2 sequences*: highly sensitive to signal abnormalities in the marrow, thanks to the myelographic effect (hypersignal of the CSF). The fleshy portion of the tumor is most often hypersignal, but hyposignals may also be present, sometimes linked to chronic bleeding (deposits of hemosiderin, a product of hemoglobin degradation). Cysts are always hypersignal.

- *Gadolinium injection in T1* is essential for the study of IMT. Contrast uptake is an indicator of tumor vascularization, and the type of gadolinium uptake (heterogeneous or homogeneous) is a key factor in the differential diagnosis of tumors such as ependymoma, hemangioblastoma or astrocytoma, heterogeneous uptake being in favor of anaplastic or malignant IMTs.

- *Axial slices*: these can be used to localize the width of the IMT in the medullary cord in relation to the ependymal canal: central (ependymoma), eccentric (astrocytoma), anterior (ependymoglial cyst), posterior or exophytic (hemangioblastoma, cavernoma), and thus help plan surgery. In some cases, flow MRI can be used to differentiate tumor cysts from syringomyelia, fat saturation (for lipoma diagnosis), flair (for edema) and tractography (to study spinal cord bundles).

- In at-risk patients or known carriers of genetic diseases such as *phacomatosis* (Neurofibromatosis: NF or Von Hippel Lindau: VHL), MRI can easily explore the entire neuraxis.

- MRI can differentiate between *non-tumoral cystic formations,* such as malformative syringomyelia, which are most often associated with a craniocervical hinge anomaly, or cavities secondary to trauma or arachnoiditis.

However informative the analysis may be, MRI cannot answer a question often asked before surgery. Is the tumour resectable? Although certain signs are suggestive of good tumor demarcation, such as homogeneous gadolinium enhancement or clear demarcation from healthy tissue on T2-weighted images, it is not possible to define radiological criteria that accurately predict the resectability or histology of IMT. A recent preliminary study [231] suggests that diffusion tensor tractography performed on 13 IMTs including 8 ependymomas, 2 lymphomas and 3 astrocytomas is capable of predicting IMT resectability and thus, imaging was classified into three types, depending on whether the medullary fiber trajectory is taken by the lesion or not, in this perspective 6/13 of lesions were considered resectable and intraoperatively 7/13 of lesions presented a cleavage plane.

As a result, the reliability of this technique is considered substantial [154].

Differential diagnosis with inflammatory and demyelinating conditions is difficult, particularly with lesions that take up little or no gadolinium. As a general rule, inflammatory and demyelinating lesions never occupy space [148]; when in doubt, close MRI scans performed a few weeks apart reveal labile lesions, leading to different radiological appearances within a few weeks or months. Tumors will never change appearance in such a short time [228]. Furthermore, in demyelinating lesions such as multiple sclerosis, are multifocal and brain MRI reveals multiple localizations [154].

Another pathology to consider is post-radiation myelopathy, a rare but potentially serious complication of radiotherapy, and occurs when the irradiation field includes the spinal cord. MRI in the acute stage shows intramedullary hypersignal on T2-weighted sequences, associated with perilesional medullary edema, and Gadolinium enhancement in around half of cases. At a later stage, the medulla appears atrophic. There appears to be no correlation between clinical manifestations and atrophy [228].

3.5.1.3. Angiography

Angiography is recommended by some surgeons before approaching certain giant hemangioblastomas for possible preoperative embolization [42].

3.5.2. Electrical examinations

With an abnormality detection rate of over 90%, PES is the leading functional diagnostic test for IMDs of all clinical presentations. An abnormality of intraspinal sensitive or motor conduction is detectable in over 60% of cervical MCI.

The study of preoperative somaesthetic and motor evoked potentials makes it possible to quantify neurological damage, assess the feasibility of intraoperative monitoring and follow its evolution postoperatively [208].

V. TREATMENT

When faced with an intramedullary tumour, it is essential to assess the risk-benefit ratio of both an intervention and a wait-and-see attitude. The diagnosis of a tumour alone does not constitute an indication for surgery.

The patient's clinical condition, radiological characteristics and tumor location are all factors to be taken into consideration in the management of IMT, on a case-by-case basis.

It is accepted that the risk of neurological deterioration is lower the smaller the preoperative deficits, and conversely, higher the poorer the preoperative condition.

Early diagnosis is vital, as already established deficits rarely recover even after complete removal of the tumour. Surgery, on the other hand, is often without severe morbidity, in which case it is often transient [26133].

As in the case of the brain, the problem arises with incidentally discovered TIMs. The principle is therefore to operate on any accessible tumour that presents a clinical and/or radiological risk of progression, or is at high risk of spontaneous bleeding.

1. SURGERY

As with any neurosurgical procedure, the first step in approaching a patient with IMD is to define the aim of the surgery, which in the long term is control or cure with preservation of neurological function.

1.1. Anesthetic considerations

The principle is to ensure good spinal cord perfusion throughout surgery.

Corticosteroid therapy: there are no recommendations, but several authors give high doses of corticosteroids before, during and after surgery [108-109]. However, Woodworth et al [263] report that a blood glucose level in excess of 170 mg/dl in the peri-operative period is a factor of poor functional prognosis.

1.2. Technical aids

The technical aids listed below make surgery increasingly risk-free, particularly in terms of neurological prognosis.

1.2.1. Microscope

Microscopes and microsurgical instruments are becoming increasingly sophisticated, and are now indispensable in the practice of IMT surgery.

The operating microscope is essential for the excision of IMTs, especially as the cleavage plane is difficult to individualize, and the tumor-moel transition zone can only be recognized under the microscope.

1.2.2. Ultrasonic surgical aspirator

The development and application of the ultrasonic aspirator has made a significant contribution to spinal cord surgery. The direct application of the high-frequency vibrating tip to tumor tissue results in cavitation, rupture and fragmentation. The fragmented tissue, soaked by irrigation fluid, is then aspirated through the hollow tip [80].

1.2.3. Ultrasound

Complementary to MRI, it is used sterile trans-durally or sub-durally. Ultrasound confirms the suitability of laminectomy or laminotomy for exposure, and helps differentiate solid tumors from associated cysts (intra-tumoral and satellite). These images can help to approximate the tumoral nature; thus ependymomas tend to be uniformly echogenic and have a central, symmetrical location in contrast to astrocytomas which are relatively iso-echogenic, eccentric and often present a heterogeneous echo (foci of calcifications or tumoral cysts) [127160-173].

Echodoppler provides hemodynamic information and determines the vascularization of certain vascular IMTs [86]. The ultrasound image is useful in planning myelotomy and approaching the tumor: if satellite cysts are present, myelotomy is started at the cyst-tumor junction, but failing this, myelotomy is performed on the largest part of the tumor where the risk of damaging the posterior cords is minimal. Finally, ultrasound helps in the radical resection of IMTs: a persistent abnormal signal or an uncollapsed intra-tumoral cyst will prompt the surgeon to continue with the excision.

1.2.4. The laser

In IMT surgery, lasers provide high-precision tumor excision with minimal trauma (thermal and mechanical) to the surrounding nerve tissue. There are different types of laser, of which carbon dioxide and Neodymium Yttrium Aluminum Garnet (Nd: YAG) are commonly used [16]. The surgeon can move the laser beam around the operating field, and the concentrated light source performs the myelotomy with minimum dispersion and extreme precision, reducing damage to the posterior cords [102]. It can dissect or vaporize firm tumor tissue, particularly lipomas, which can be reduced with little bleeding, to dimensions difficult to achieve with other techniques and [120].

1.2.5. Monitoring evoked potentials

Intraoperative neurophysiological monitoring has become a standard procedure to optimize tumor resection and minimize neurological morbidity [12]. Its use requires both neurophysiological expertise on the part of the surgeon and the presence of a monitoring team capable of handling the necessary equipment.

The role of evoked potentials is to detect imminent, reversible and/or repairable damage intraoperatively, alerting the surgeon to adapt his or her operative strategy to prevent postoperative neurological deficits.

Initially, only PES was monitored, but it reflected little or no real-time functional integrity of the motor pathways, with false negatives [124]. Combined monitoring of PES and PEM has become almost systematic, as there is a possibility of selective injury to either somato-sensory or motor pathways [222].

1.2.5.1. Anesthesia

Particularly in EMP, anesthesia is maintained by constant infusion of propofol (100-150g/kg/min) and fentanyl (1g/kg/h). Nitrous oxide should not exceed 50%. Rapid-acting muscle relaxants are used only for tracheal intubation, and should be avoided thereafter, along with halogens and curares [221].

1.2.5.2. Somatosensory evoked potentials

PES explores the lemniscal proprioceptive pathways running along the posterior cords of the medulla, providing quasi-continuous monitoring. Stimulation is performed on the median nerve at the wrist and the posterior tibial nerve at the ankle, and cortical and subcortical PES recordings are collected via corkscrew electrodes inserted into the scalp (Fig. 17a) [144bis-204].

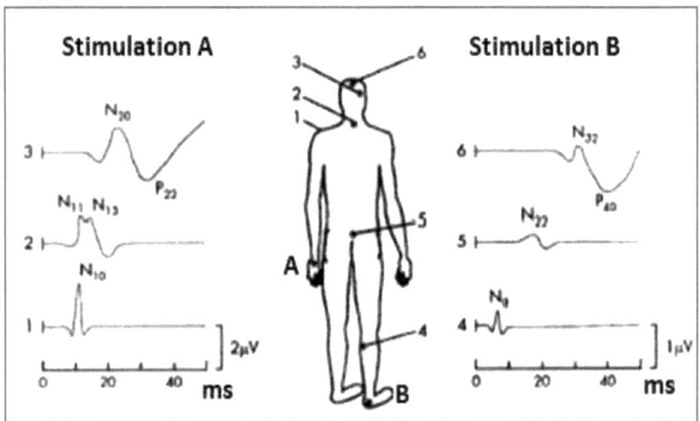

Fig. 17a: Somatosensory evoked potentials. **Center,** locations of stimulation and stepped collection points. **Left:** median nerve stimulation at wrist (A), staged collection at brachial plexus (1), 7ème cervical vertebra (2), and lateral parietal region (3). **Right:** stimulation of the posterior tibial nerve at the ankle (B), staged collection at the popliteal fossa (4), lumbar region (5), and central parietal region (6). The denomination of the various response components corresponds to their polarity (N, negative; P, positive) followed by their mean latency (expressed in ms). Peripheral sensitive conduction velocities are calculated from responses 1 and 4,

and central conduction times by the differences N20 - N13, and P40 - N22. [144 bis].

1.2.5.2. Motor evoked potentials

Motor evoked potentials (MEPs) follow the pyramidal motor pathway, but only allow discontinuous or "on-demand" monitoring. The sensitivity of MEPs in relation to postoperative motor deficits is close to 100%, and their specificity is of the order of 90%. PEMs are therefore a good reflection of "clinical reality" [137]. They are obtained by transcranial electrical stimulation of the motor cortex. A technique based on the use of "trains of stimulations" allows EMG recording of muscle responses, while "single stimulations" allow epidural D-waves to be recorded downstream of the surgical site (Fig.17b).

1.2.5.3. Interest

Monitoring enables us to locate the posterior median sulcus and, above all, to detect conduction anomalies on the PEM and PES.

➢ *Locating the posterior median sulcus*: wire-mounted electrodes are placed transversely across the posterior cord to record PES waves. The median sulcus is located midway between two PES amplitude peaks on either side, where responses are absent or weakest [171-204].

➢ Signs or alarm criteria: these appear when modifications are made to registrations, PES and PEM.

• PES: A 50% decrease in amplitude and/or a 10% prolongation in latency are considered significant, and should prompt a change in myelotomy location. Overall, the preservation of PES is strongly recommended; however, its loss during myelotomy is not a criterion for discontinuing surgery [28-138].

• PEM: These recordings provide specific, semi-quantitative

information on the functional integrity of the fast conducting fibers of the corticospinal bundle. They are essential for establishing warning criteria and predicting prognosis [59-81-222]. Any significant increase in latency or net decrease in amplitude should prompt the patient to suspend surgery, identify the aggressive gesture and adjust the surgical procedure.

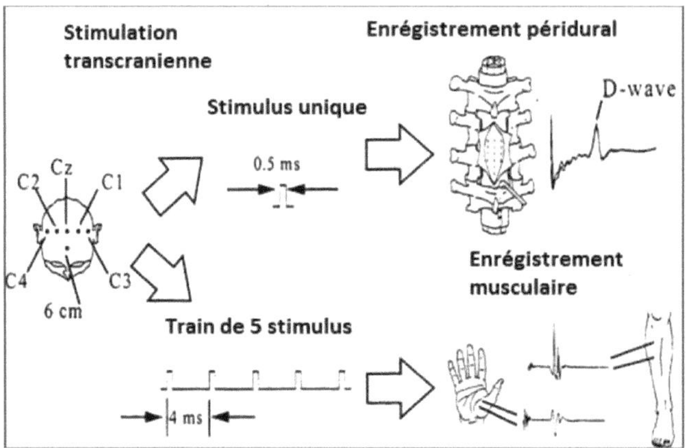

Fig.17b: Motor evoked potentials: **Left**: schematic illustration showing electrode positioning for transcranial electrical stimulation of the motor cortex. **Top right**: diagram of epidural electrode positioning downstream of the lesion for monitoring the signal (D-wave) passing through the surgical site after a single stimulus. **Bottom right**: recording of mMEPs distal to the distal muscles after a short train of electrical stimulation. [222].

1.3. The TIM approach

The approach to IMT is almost exclusively posterior, and generally in the prone position. Every precaution must be taken to keep the abdomen free to facilitate venous return, in order to limit epidural venous bleeding.

For cervical and cervico-dorsal tumors, the semi-sitting position, for experienced and familiar teams of anesthetists, could be very comfortable for the surgeon, as it offers considerable advantages, in particular a clean operating field easy to maintain at all times by simple irrigation, without having to resort to frequent aspiration, an additional source of spinal cord trauma.

The level of the lesion is identified intraoperatively under fluoroscopic control, or sometimes beforehand by standard spinal X-rays, centered on the lesion site.

The skin incision is median, then, once all the vertebral arches are exposed, the laminectomy or laminotomy (Fig. 18) is performed using the rodents or craniotome. Epidural fat and veins are often compressed and displaced laterally by TIM; and veins only begin to bleed after volumetric reduction of the tumour.

Sometimes a minimally invasive approach is sufficient for small lateralized IMTs [20-155-190]. Yasargil et al [268] used hemilaminectomies to approach hemangioblastomas. The advantage of this approach is the preservation of the posterior ligaments on the midline and the blades on the opposite side.

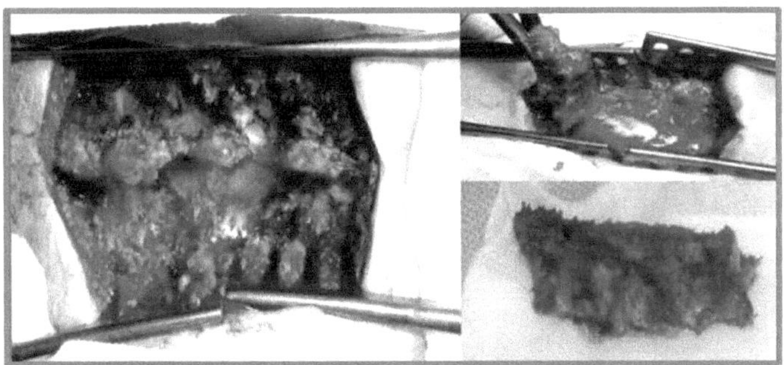

Fig. 18: Exposure of posterior arches and laminotomy.

The dura mater is opened on the midline and its edges suspended laterally under tension, thus maintaining exposure of the medulla and at the same time autostatic epidural hemostasis (Fig.19).

The arachnoid membrane and its septa are carefully dissected to avoid damage to small vessels and strain on the medulla.

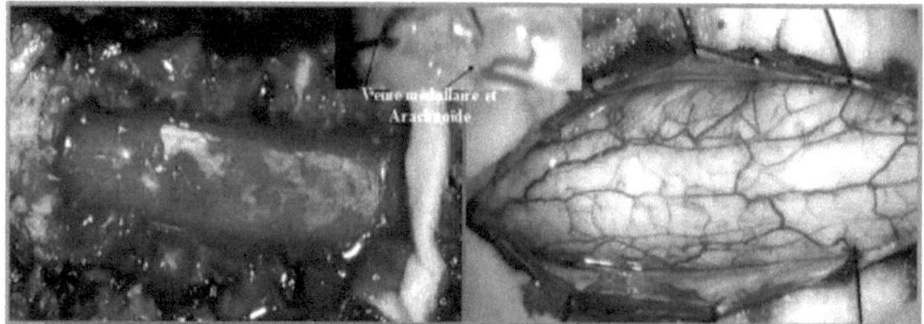

Fig. 19: Exposure, opening and suspension of the mother ure under the operating microscope.

1.3. Tumor removal (Fig. 19)

The spinal cord is inspected for signs of tumor focus, i.e. discoloration, swelling, torsion, bleeding or tortuous venous appearance. Ultrasound at this stage is of considerable help in verifying that exposure is sufficient and adequate before beginning myelotomy [127]. The latter is performed on the posterior median sulcus, which may be difficult to determine due to distortion of the posterior aspect of the medulla (Fig. 20. 22). In this case, the groove above and below the tumour and/or the posterior roots on either side must be identified.

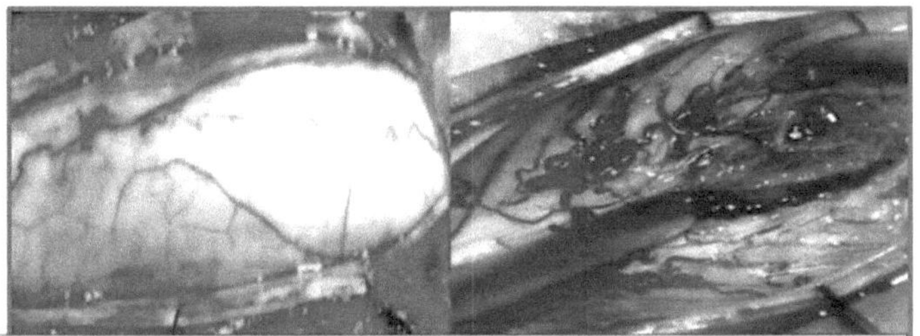

Fig. 20: Posterior aspect of the spinal cord.

Coagulation of the medullary surface should be avoided, as this could lead to significant sensory problems.

While myelotomy is generally performed over the entire extent of the tumor mass [245], some authors prefer intermittent myelotomies, performed using a diamond knife or micro-scissors, or even the laser to cut the pie-mother [34] ; the opening is completed by simple separation of the cords using micro-instruments, which makes the term myelotomy inappropriate, as it is much more a separation, since a thin fibrous structure to which small vessels converge, and which can serve as a good landmark for the surgeon, separates the marrow into two halves [72]. Next, the edges of the myelotomy are suspended from the dura mater with 6-0 suture to keep the medulla open and minimize its manipulation during tumor removal, and to protect the lateral surfaces of the spinal cord from injury (Fig. 21). This may subsequently facilitate determination of the cleavage plane once the tumor has been emptied, with the exception of hemangioblastoma, which must be removed as a monobloc [108-228].

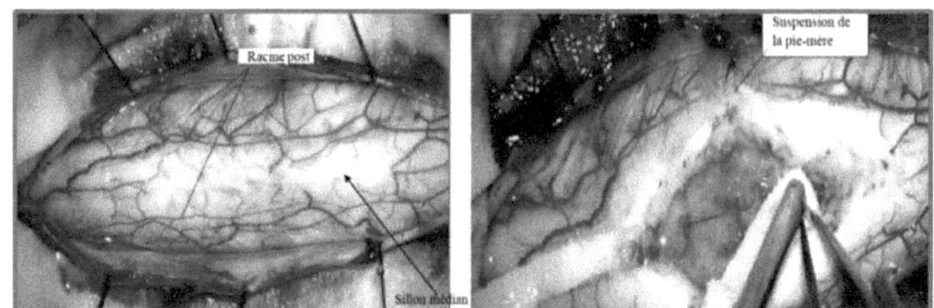

Fig. 21: Suspension of the myelotomy and evidence of the lesion

Depending on the consistency of the tumour and its vascularization, volumetric reduction is achieved step by step by coagulation and morcellation, or by CUSA and, in some cases, laser [102]. Once tumour retraction has been achieved, dissection is started by following the cleavage plane all the way around (Fig. 23), with the exception of infiltrating IMTs, where it is necessary to remain as far inside the tumour as possible, and to stop excision once the transition zone between tumour tissue and medullary cord has become uncertain.

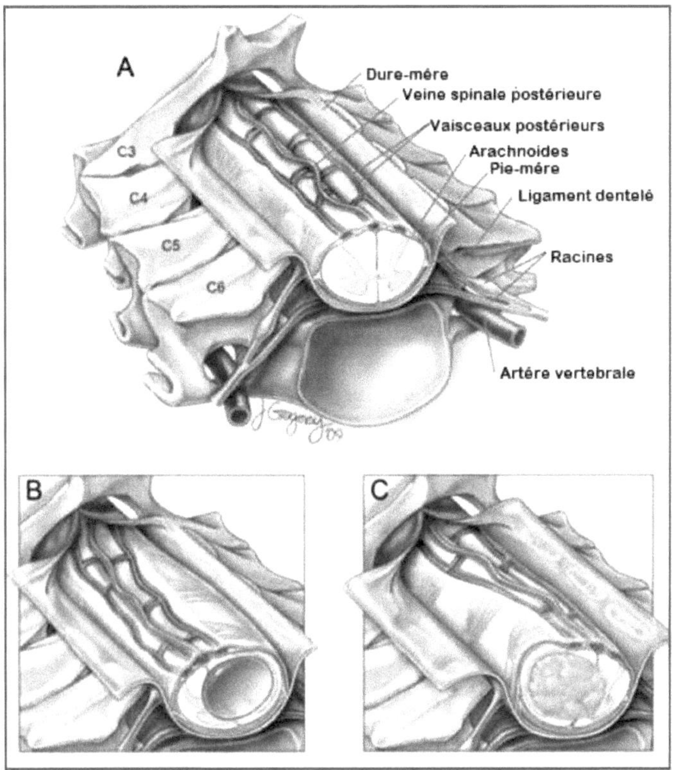

Fig. 22: Illustration of the anatomy of the dorsal surface of the spinal cord. **(A):** Normal medulla with median sulcus in the middle of the posterior columns. **(B):** Rotation and widening of the medulla secondary to a syrinx. **(C):** Distortion of the medial sulcus secondary to a TIM. [58].

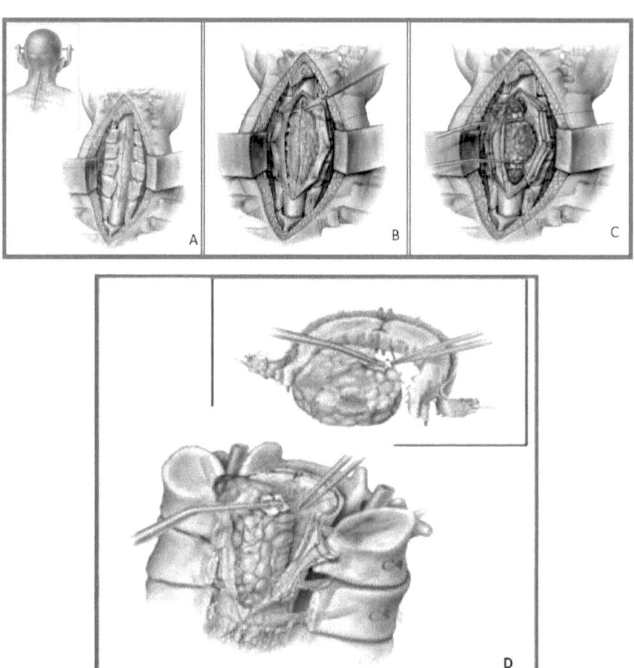

Fig. 23: TIM resection technique. **(A):** Laminectomy. **(B):** Median opening and suspension of the dura mater, then access to the posterior aspect of the medulla by dissecting the arachnoid. The myelotomy is median. **(C):** Slight traction on the dura mater to facilitate dissection of the tumor rim in the middle and at the poles. **(D) :** In hemangioblastoma, ependymoma and pilocytic astrocytoma, the cleavage plane between tumor and nerve tissue is generally individualizable. After completing the dissection laterally and at the tumor poles, the ventral part of the tumor is dissected and then resected by exerting gentle traction, the feeder vessels are coagulated and cut. [11] [85].

Whatever the nature of the tumour, the cleavage plane between the tumour and the healthy tissue is decisive for the entire exeresis. The absence of a cleavage plane should prompt caution, especially if the macroscopic appearance and/or extemporaneous histology are in favour of a malignant and/or infiltrative IMT.

In vascular lesions such as hemangioblastoma and cavernoma,

coagulation of the tumor surface opens up the cleavage plane. In patients who have been irradiated, a gliotic plane has been created by radiotherapy, which can make dissection and identification of a correct cleavage plane very difficult; the possible presence of a polar syrinx helps to clearly delineate tumor boundaries [22-78]. Old bleeding facilitates dissection, whereas fresh bleeding may make individualization of the cleavage plane difficult or impossible, and in this case, radical resection should not be attempted.

Care must be taken to identify tumour feeders that need to be coagulated and sectioned, particularly in ependymomas where important feeder arteries arise from the anterior spinal artery. Dissection must minimize any excessive tension on these feeder vessels to avoid any compromise to this important artery. This is often achieved by changing the dissection zone from left to right, top to bottom and *vice versa*. Intraoperative ultrasound is a valuable aid in assessing the quality of excision [37-209]. As a rule, the majority of polar cysts are non-tumoral and require simple drainage [165].

At the end of the procedure, most benign non-invasive tumours are completely removed. Careful haemostasis is ensured by simple cotton swabbing and surgicel, which is subsequently removed, as coagulation of the operating bed is not highly recommended. The piea mater is closed with separate stitches of very fine thread, and the dura mater is hermetically sutured if necessary, with dural plasty for enlargement.

In the case of laminotomy, the osteoligamentous block is put back in place and fixed with non-ferromagnetic mini-plates [133], while taking care not to compress the marrow; then the musculoaponeurotic and cutaneous planes are tightly closed to prevent CSF leakage.

1.4. Two-stage surgery

Reported for the first time by Elsberg [103] in 1910, two-stage surgery is now finding its way into low-grade, infiltrating and extensive astrocytomas. The myelotomy left open in the first stage of surgery will allow spontaneous delivery of tumor tissue by intra-parenchymal pressure, making dissection and removal of the tumor easier in the 2ème stage.

1.5. Iterative surgery

In cases of recurrence, epidural scar dissection is difficult, and the principle is to begin dissection in a healthy area, upstream or downstream of the first opening, enlarging the laminectomy to identify the healthy dura mater.

If the previous operation involved a laminotomy, exposure of the dura mater is easier. As the areas of adhesion to the posterior cord are generally just below the suture line, the dura mater is consequently opened laterally, and its suspension must be cautious due to adhesions to the cord and its vessels. As far as possible, the arachnoid is opened separately. In some recurrences, it is even difficult to distinguish between the arachnoid and the surface of the spinal cord. The posterior median groove is located midway between the posterior roots. Depending on the ultrasonographic images, it may be necessary to extend the myelotomy to complete the myelotomy.

complete resection. The dural closure will be performed with an enlargement plasty to prevent the formation of additional adhesions.

2. ADJUVANT THERAPY

The treatment of choice for TIM remains surgical, aiming for complete excision. Biopsy followed by radiotherapy and/or chemotherapy is no longer an option for benign TIM.

2.1. Radiotherapy

High-grade IMTs (WHO grades III and IV) tend to have a high rate of local and distant recurrence throughout the neuraxis, prompting several authors to advocate craniospinal radiotherapy, which can improve both local tumor control and overall survival [1-4176-114-135-150-232-240-272].

If complete exeresis cannot be achieved, radiotherapy has been recommended by some authors for ependymomas [40-111-216-232] and astrocytomas [77-101-111], while Chigasaki, Epstein, Roux et al [40-73-216] deny any beneficial effect for astrocytomas and Mork, McCormick et al [165-180] for ependymomas. It seems that effective doses in excess of 40 Gy are at the same time toxic to medullary tissue [84].

The efficacy of radiosurgery on benign IMT has not yet been established. Ryu et al [203-218] presented a series of seven patients with ependymomas and hemangioblastomas: two improved, four remained stable and one patient died after a survival of 2 years.

Colnat-Coulbois et al [47] reported a case of intramedullary cystic pilocytic astrocytoma treated by surgery and 2 intracavitary injections of rhenium 186, and achieved stabilization of the cyst, with minor side effects and dramatic improvement in neurological deficits.

2.2. Chemotherapy

The role of chemotherapy in high-grade tumors has yet to be determined [13-181]. Chemotherapy as an adjunct to surgical treatment of IMT is of interest in the paediatric population due to the deleterious effects of radiotherapy [17]. Chamberlain reported the results of a prospective study of 10 ependymoma recurrences treated with oral etoposide. Control MRI was performed every 8 weeks between cycles of chemotherapy. After the 1er cycle of etoposide, 3 patients showed disease progression, 2 patients showed a partial response and 5 patients were stable. The median duration of stability was 15 months [36].

In 1997, Allen et al [6] presented the results of a prospective study of the "8-in-1" protocol in 13 children operated on for high-grade intramedullary astrocytomas enrolled in the Children's Cancer Group (CCG) protocol 945. At 5 years, 7 children were still alive, 5 with stable disease and 2 cured. Although the results were favorable in comparison with other studies, it was impossible to credit this chemotherapy protocol alone with its good results.

3. RESULTS

Intraoperative electrophysiological monitoring is a very useful tool for optimizing the quality of excision and reducing the risk of serious neurological complications (paraplegia, tetraplegia) [164-221-222].

3.1. Quality of excision

Neuroradiological assessment of the rate of resection is often difficult in the immediate postoperative period due to variations in gadolinium uptake of remodels, which are difficult to differentiate from tumor remnants [237].

With the introduction of the operating microscope, the rate of complete resection (all histologies combined) increased significantly. For Yang et al [265], resection was total in 69%, subtotal in 17.8% and partial in 13.2%; for Klekamp et al [133], resection was total in 53%, subtotal in 32% and the remaining 15% underwent decompression and biopsy or cystostomy with or without drainage.

Total excision should never be a goal in itself, especially when there is no cleavage plane, particularly in infiltrating gliomas, and/or when the surgeon lacks experience.

3.2. Clinical results

Immediate post-operative outcome depends primarily on pre-operative neurological status, tumour location and surgeon experience, but is little influenced by histology. The quality of excision has little influence on short-term postoperative outcome. Klekamp et al [133] found transient neurological worsening in 44% of operated IMTs. The return to pre-operative status lasted from a few days to a few months. The cause of this aggravation was attributed to edema or altered spinal cord hemodynamics.

In the series by Sandalcioglu et al [224], around two-thirds of patients improved or remained stable, while the remaining one-third worsened. Thoracic IMT is associated with higher morbidity. Pain may subside after excision, while dysesthesias generally remain unchanged, and sensory deficits tend to worsen [133-224].

The quality of excision may play an indirect role in long-term results, due to tumor evolution and growth, which will lead to poorer clinical results later on. According to Yang et al [265], improvement in neurological function is observed in 70% of patients, *status quo* in 19.5%, worsening in 4% and 6.3% death due to tumor recurrence.

3.3. Mortality

Surgical mortality in the first month ranges from 1.1 to 6.3%, the cause being mainly related to respiratory disorders [133-265].

3.4. Complications

Complications attributed to IMT surgery can be divided into early and late complications.

3.4.1. Short-term complications

According to the National Inpatient Sample (NIS), the complication rate is 17.5% [199]. The most frequently reported complications are urinary or renal, postoperative hemorrhage or hematoma, pulmonary complications, CSF fistula, wound infection, spinal cord edema and acute psychosis [48-79-133-224].

3.4.2. Late complications

Late complications include spinal instability and post-surgical myelopathy.

- *Instability*: this complication is more frequent in poor pre-operative functional scores, thoraco-lumbar locations and in pediatric age [166 -167-168-267]. Post-laminectomy deformity is observed in 24% to 40% of children operated on for TIM [109-157-247] and in 66% of children for Jallo et al [117], 35% of whom required stabilization. Klekamp et al [133] found none in a mainly adult series. Blade reinsertion with mini-plates is strongly recommended, if not mandatory, particularly in children [i0-i8i-239]. Moreover, spinal atrophy and muscle denervation alone can induce instability and sometimes even aggravation of vertebral deformities already present prior to surgery.

- *Myelopathy*: a significant number of patients develop a postoperative dysesthetic syndrome, characterized by unpleasant sensations, burning and pain; sometimes progressive neurological deterioration by myelopathy in the absence of tumor recurrence can be observed [133]. The etiology of this myelopathy is unclear, and probably related to several factors, Greenwood [91] having attributed it to gliosis, Peker [201] to the extent of the myelotomy; whereas for Hoshimaru [107], Raco et al [206] it is the post-fixed medulla following scarring fibrosis of the arachnoid that is to blame.

3.5. Tumor recurrence and clinical relapse

In addition to tumor recurrence, other mechanisms can lead to postoperative clinical deterioration.

Overall, tumor recurrence rates are 24% and 26% after 5 and 10 years respectively [90]. Klekamp et al [133] report that after complete resection, local recurrence rates are 3%, 8% and 13% after 1, 5 and 10 years respectively; and that complete resection of low-grade malignant IMT with cervical and high thoracic localization are factors contributing to a low recurrence rate. The difference between local recurrence of benign and malignant tumours is significant: in benign tumours, the recurrence rate is 9% and 18% after 1 and 5 years respectively, whereas in malignant tumours it is 44% and 68% respectively [90]. On the other hand, factors predisposing to long-term clinical stabilization are complete excision, high tumor location and absence of post-fixed marrow [133].

5. SURVIVAL

Median progression-free survival correlates with the quality of excision and histology (Fig. 17); thus, MIPTs with a cleavage plane, benign tumours or low-grade malignancies such as hemangioblatoma and ependymoma II, have the longest median progression-free survival (PFS) [83].

Klekamp et al [133] found a postoperative survival rate of 87% at 1 year, 76% at 5 years, and 73% at 10 years. His analysis found that low-grade histology, absence of recurrence, absence of arachnoiditis, a good pre-operative functional score and a long pre-operative history were associated with long survival.

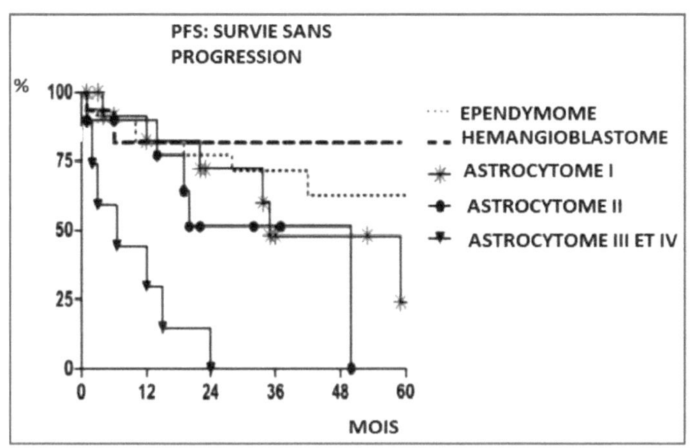

Fig. 24: PFS as a function of tumour type[83].

VI. PATHOLOGICAL ENTITIES

In order to gain a better understanding of IMTs, this chapter looks at the various histological entities, with their different diagnostic and therapeutic aspects. Ependymomas, astrocytomas, hemangioblanstomas, cavernomas, metastases, harmatomas, melanocytomas and many others will be discussed in turn.

1. EPENDYMOMAS

Ependymoma is a tumor of the central nervous system whose essential component consists of cells derived from the ependyma of the central medullary canal, first described in 1863 by Virchow and defined as a distinct histological entity by Bailey and Cushing in 1926 [153].

Ependymomas are the most common IMTs, most of which are benign and well-limited, allowing complete resection without major functional worsening [12].

1.1. Epidemiology

According to the CBTRUS (Central Brain Tumor Registry of the United States), the incidence of ependymomas is 0.06/100000/year, representing approximately 45% of IMTs and over 60% of intramedullary glial tumors [35-228].

In adults, IMT is the most common (50-60%), with a peak age between 42.8 and 46 years, and a slight male preponderance in 55-67% of cases [2 -22-141-228].

1.2. Clinical semiology

The onset of clinical signs is usually slow and insidious. Diagnosis time is often long, greater than or equal to 1 year in 56% of cases, and ranges from 30 to 40 months [22-96-133-141]. Worsening is progressive, but brutal forms have been reported [2].

There is no clinical differentiation between ependymomas and other slowly progressing intramedullary processes. The onset of clinical signs appears to be more insidious and slower than in astrocytomas.

The clinical picture is characterized by varying degrees of pain, sensory-motor disorders and sphincter disorders.

1.3. MRI imaging

Classically, the lesion appears on MRI (Fig.21) as an enlargement of the spinal cord, clearly visible on T1 sequences. The tumor is often centrally located and well limited. The most consistent feature is hyperintense lesions on T2 sequences. In T1, the tumor's behavior is less regular; it is most often isointense (70%) or slightly hypointense (27%), but may in rare cases be hyperintense (3%). After gadolinium injection, contrast enhancement appears to be 100% systematic [178-246] and 80% for Brotchi [27]. For Sun et al [246], contrast enhancement is homogeneous in 75% of cases and heterogeneous in 25%, while Miyazawa and Mork [178-180] consider the type of enhancement to be variable.

A cyst is very often associated with the fleshy portion and found in 90% of Miyazawa, 61% of Sun and 54% of Chang's cases [38-178-246]. The cyst may be intratumoral, uniolar or bipolar. The cyst is always hypointense in T1 and hyperintense in T2. Miyazawa reports that in

65% of cases, the intracystic signal is different from that of the CSF [178].

Overall, the lesion appears to be perfectly circumscribed in 70-80% of cases. The existence of intratumoral haemorrhagic stigmata and a hypointense area at both poles of the fleshy portion have been considered radiological signs in favour of an ependymoma (cuff sign) [27]. The lesion is most often located in the cervical spine in 41.5 to 92% of cases, followed by the thoracic spine in 8 to 28% of cases, and more rarely in the lumbar spine in 0 to 17% of cases [2-178-246].

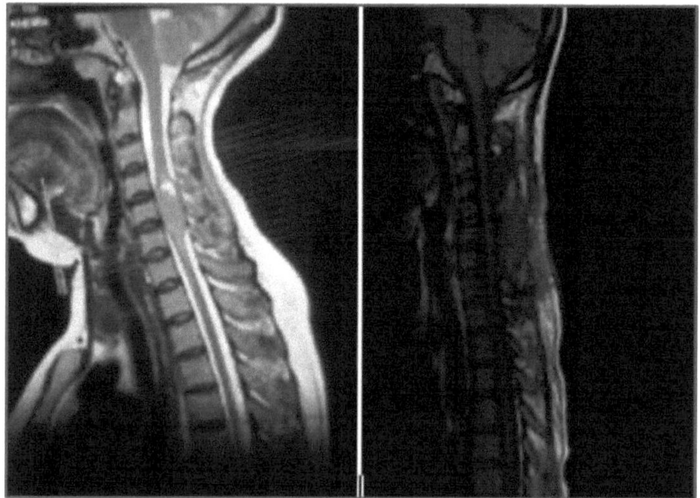

Fig .25. Sagittal-section MRI of a cervical ependymoma, in preoperative T2 and postoperative T1 sequences.

1.4. Histology

The WHO classification [153] recognizes three grades of ependymoma:

- *Grade I*: myxopapillary ependymoma (excluded from IMT).
- *Grade II*: classic intermediate, cellular, papillary, clear-cell and

tanycytic ependymomas (all WHO stage II).

- *Grade III*: anaplastic ependymoma.

Macroscopically, ependymomas vary in color from brown to purplish [79]. Unlike astrocytomas, these lesions are well-demarcated, have a good cleavage plane and are frequently associated with peri- or intratumoral cysts [18]. Histologically (Fig. 22), classical ependymoma is characterized by pseudorosette formations and true aligned ependymal rosettes; mitotic figures are rare. Anaplastic ependymoma is characterized by hypercellularity, elevated mitotic index, microvascular proliferation and occasional necrosis. Published series include very rare malignant ependymomas 2.4 to 3.33% [2-27].

In molecular biology, genetic abnormalities in sporadic ependymomas include mutation of the NF2 gene, loss of chromosome 22 and loss of 17p [197-257]. In a recent study, Ebert et al [66] found allelic loss of 10q, 22q and somatic mutations of NF2. Ependymomas are seen more frequently in NF2 [64].

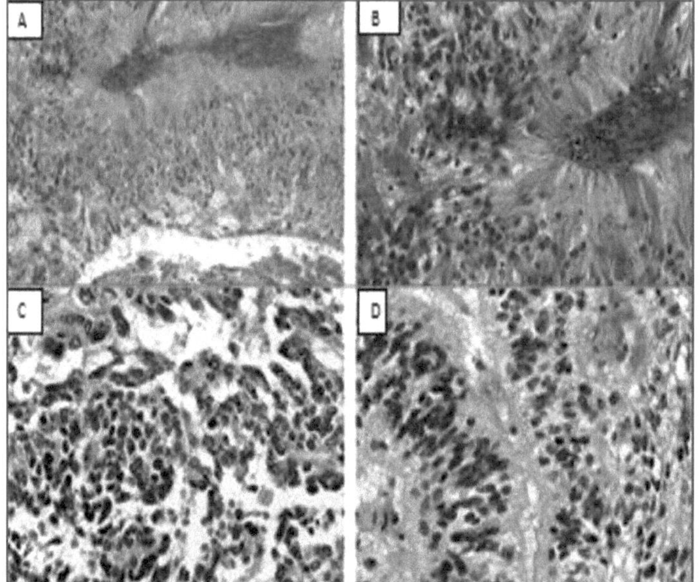

Fig. 26: Histopathology of ependymomas. **A.B**: Ependymoma II with perivascular pseudorosettes. **C.D**: Grade III anaplastic ependymoma with rich cell proliferation, poorly differentiated, and high mitotic activity. [22].

1.5. Treatments and results

Ependymoma is the surgical IMT par excellence, and the better the neurological status, the better the results.

1.5.1. Surgery

The treatment of choice is complete microsurgical excision, which is possible in 80-97% of cases [2-22-29-85-96-107-133]. Myelotomy should allow exposure of both poles of the lesion and inspection of the cystic wall, but should not extend further. Exeresis can be performed as a monobloc if the ependymoma is small, but it is preferable to perform debulking before any attempt at dissection.

The ependymoma is often well limited, especially if associated with a satellite cyst. The cleavage plane is almost always present; if not, it should be sought, and if not, it may be a malignant ependymoma. The color is purplish, if not brownish, and the wall is generally firm and easy to grasp; however, the friable contents are easy to pick up by the CUSA [27].

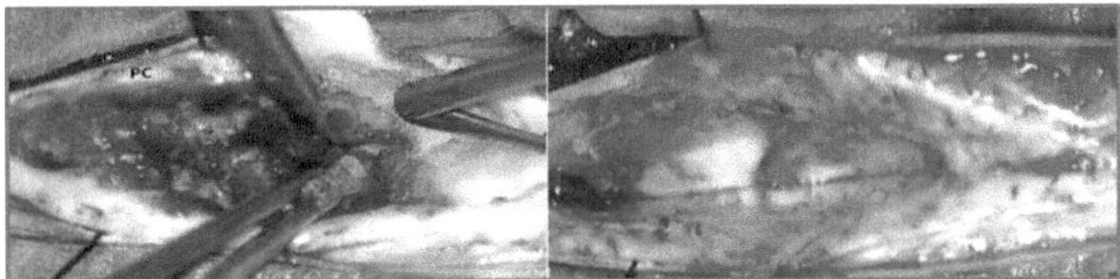
Fig. 27: Operative view of an ependymoma II with a good cleavage plane (CP) allowing total exeresis.

1.5.2. Chemotherapy

There is no evidence to support the use of chemotherapy in the initial management of ependymomas, but various molecules have been introduced into the therapeutic armamentarium for inoperable and/or already-irradiated recurrences, and appear to give interesting results, notably Etoposide, Carboplatin and Imatinib [36-76-259].

1.5.3. Radiotherapy

In a retrospective cohort of 26 patients who underwent subtotal excision, Gavin et al [85] found no statistical difference in terms of PFS between those who underwent radiotherapy and those who remained without. Given the excellent long-term results in terms of local recurrence and survival rate after surgery alone, there is a consensus not to recommend postoperative radiotherapy for ependymomas, even after incomplete resection; rather, a second operation should be attempted than proposing radiotherapy [133]. At present, radiotherapy is reserved only for patients with malignant ependymomas in the absence of surgical revision possibilities [27-149].

1.5.4. Results

The rate of complete excision varies between 69% and 97%. Patients improved in 10 to 43%, stabilized in 25 to 74.4% and worsened in 13.5 to 37% of cases [2-22-27-96-107-133-228-233]. Aghakhani et al [2], analyzing pain in greater detail, report complete disappearance in 64.8% of cases, improvement in 3.7%, stabilization in 24.1% and worsening in 7.4%. Survival rates at 5 and 10 years are 97% and 91% respectively, with a PFS of 75% at 10 years [38]. For Bostrom [22], the PFS is 97% at 5 years if total excision and 57% if subtotal.

The recurrence rate after complete resection is between 0 and 1.16%. In the case of incomplete resections, the evolution of the remnant remains fairly rare, with a recurrence rate of around 20%, whether or not postoperative radiotherapy is performed [222-133-149-259].

Even after total excision, long-term recurrence is possible, hence the importance of rigorous, prolonged postoperative clinical and radiological monitoring (18 years after the initial surgery) [27-228].

1.5.6. Complications

Intra- or peri-operative mortality ranges from 0% to 3.2%. All authors describe a period of postoperative aggravation, often transient, which improves in 6 to 24 weeks; it mainly concerns deep sensitivity, dysesthesia and paresthesia [2 -27-133].

The complication rate is 34% for Kucia [141] and is infectious (pneumopathy, urinary tract infection, meningitis), decubitus (phlebitis, pulmonary embolism, bedsore) and healing (dehiscence and leakage of CSF).

2. ASTROCYTOMAS

Astrocytomas are the most common IMTs in children, and second only to ependymomas in adults. The vast majority of astrocytomas are solitary. However, in NF patients, astrocytomas may be associated with other spinal tumors. Unlike ependymomas, astrocytomas are infiltrative; with the exception of pilocytic astrocytomas, total excision is difficult and perilous due to the rarity of the cleavage plane. The life expectancy of patients with astrocytomas is not good, even when the lesion is of low-grade malignancy [24-108-200].

2.1. Epidemiology

Astrocytomas are rare tumors, accounting for around a third of all spinal cord gliomas. Although they rank second in prevalence after ependymomas in adults, they are the most common in children, and are 10 times less common than cerebral astrocytomas.

The mean age at diagnosis is 29 years [7]. In Fischer's series [79], there is a predominance of males, with a sex ratio of 1.7, and 29% of cases are pediatric. In a recent paediatric series of 29 cases reported by Scheinemann et al [227], the predominance is also male, with a sex ratio of 2.6.

2.2. Semiology

There is a clear difference between the history of low-grade and high-grade astrocytomas, as the latter have a shorter history. Diagnosis time varies between 1 month and 4 years, with an average of 9 months [116-225-227].

Rachialgia with or without radicular pain at tumor level are the most common initial symptoms, while lower limb weakness and sensory disturbances are the symptoms that bring patients to the point of clinical and diagnostic evaluation. Vesico- sphincter disorders are late symptoms, but are sometimes present at the time of surgery. Scheinemann et al [227] stress the non-specificity of clinical signs in small children, whereas in older children pain, kyphoscoliosis and weakness of both lower limbs are the major symptoms.

The speed with which symptoms and signs progress correlates fairly well with histological grade, with the exception of certain astrocytomas which may present with an acute picture following tumor bleeding, or small children who may present with acute torticollis [227].

2.3. MRI

On T1 sequences, the tumor presents a hypointense signal, and on T2 sequences, the fleshy portion of the tumor is most often hypersignal; but hyposignals may also exist, sometimes related to chronic bleeding (hemosiderin deposits). Cysts are always hypersignal.

In the majority of cases, gadolinium injection reveals contrast, of variable homogeneity (Fig.23), and enables clear delineation of the fleshy tumor portion from the surrounding marrow and adjacent cysts.

The differential diagnosis of an astrocytoma involves metastases, inflammatory lesions (sarcoidosis, demyelinating disease), infections such as bilharzia and finally vascular lesions [148].

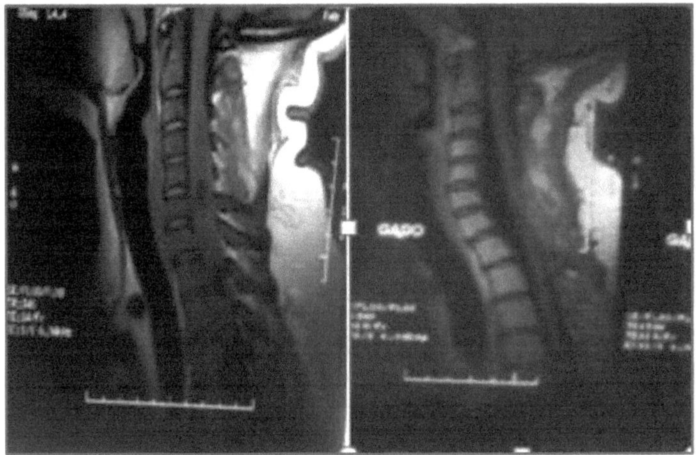

Fig. 28: Sagittal T1 gado MRI of a cervico-dorsal astrocytoma II with total exeresis

2.4. Neuropathology

These tumors developed from astrocytic cells in the spinal cord are classified according to the same WHO criteria used for cerebral astrocytomas, where grade is a good prognostic factor [35-48].

- *Grade I*: pilocytic astrocytoma.
- *Grade II*: fibrillary astrocytoma.
- *Grade III*: anaplastic astrocytoma.
- *Grade IV*: glioblastoma multiforme.

The first two entities are low-grade malignancies, accounting for 75-90% of astrocytomas.

Macroscopically, they are classically gray tumors. Their main characteristic is that they are relatively infiltrative tumors. With the exception of pilocytic astrocytomas, which are easy to individualize, these lesions generally lack a cleavage plane, making them more difficult to remove. Astrocytomas are often associated with tumour cysts, either purely intratumoral or polar [79-117-137].

Microscopically (Fig.24), pilocytic astrocytomas are characterized by elongated cells with a cytoplasm containing Rosenthal fibers and eosinophilic granular bodies. Grades II, as their name suggests, have a more fibrillar composition, while grades III and IV are identified by the presence of hypercellularity, anaplasia and high mitotic activity.

Astrocytomas usually localize in one part of the medulla and rarely involve a large area to become "holocord or pan-medullary astrocytoma". The tumor may grow diffusely with blurred boundaries with adjacent normal tissue, and may extend along nerve roots.

An important feature is the presence of satellite syrinxes, which occur in around 40% of astrocytomas. These syrinxes are more frequent in low-grade than in high-grade astrocytomas, more rostral than caudal, and less present in astrocytomas than in ependymomas [223-240].

In molecular biology, there have been no specific studies of genetic mutations in sporadic intramedullary astrocytomas; however, by transposition, it is likely that some, if not all, of the genetic alterations described in intracerebral astrocytomas play a role in the progression of intramedullary astrocytoma.

Three transitions have been studied as a paradigm 1) astrocyte to astrocytoma, 2) astrocytoma to anaplastic astrocytoma, and 3) anaplastic astrocytoma to glioblastoma [104-105]. In the first transition, the p53 mutation and losses of chromosomes 17p and 22q have been implicated; from astrocytoma to anaplastic astrocytoma, the genetic defect involves the retinoblastoma gene mutation, loss of chromosomes 9p, 13q, 19q and deletion of the p16 gene [256], and from anaplastic astrocytoma to glioblastoma, loss of chromosome 10 and amplification of the EGF gene receptor [151]. Several studies have identified the PTEN gene as one of the candidates for chromosome loss in glioblastoma [198]. Solitary astrocytomas are most commonly seen in NF1 [64].

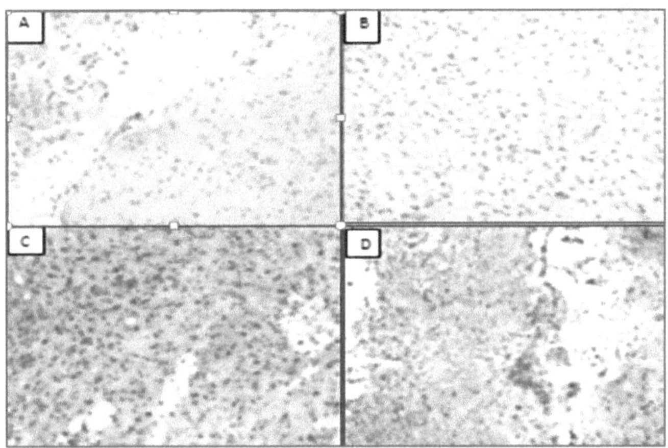

Fig. 29: Histopathology of astrocytomas. **A.** Pilocytic astrocytoma: elongated biphasic cells with Rosenthal fibers and microcysts. **B.** Grade II astrocytoma marked by moderate hypercelularity and nuclear pleomorphism. **C** Anaplastic astrocytoma III marked by cell proliferation, nuclear pleomorphism and mitotic activity. **D.** Glioblastoma grade IV: Same as grade III with endotheliocapillary proliferation. [212].

2.5. Treatment and prognosis

Astrocytoma surgery remains a formidable challenge for the surgeon, while adjuvant treatment, despite its broad indication, remains uncertain.

2.5.1: surgery

In general, astrocytomas are considered to be infiltrative tumors, so the search for a cleavage plane involves considerable risk and may even be outright impossible [108]; however, according to some authors [75], some astrocytomas present a cleavage plane allowing complete resection, using dissection techniques similar to ependymoma.

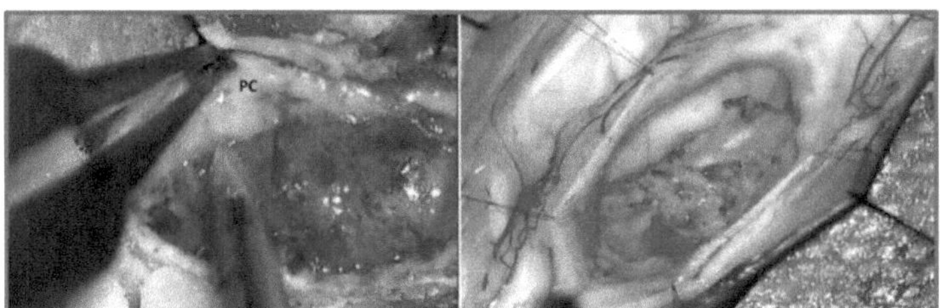

Fig. 30: Surgical view of an astrocytoma II with cleavage plane (CP) allowing total exeresis equivalent to ependymoe II.

The strategy for excision is to start in the middle of the tumour (from the inside), and CUSA is ideal for reducing tumour mass [71-116]. Tumor vascularization is not regularly ensured by the anterior spinal artery as in ependymomas. Whatever the dissection technique, there is a real danger of creating a false cleavage plane. Only macroscopic data on pathological tissue consistency and color can be used as guidelines for tumour reduction and further excision. The latter should be interrupted whenever the cleavage plane is not found and/or the tumoral appearance merges with normal bone marrow tissue [17-71108-245].

In pan-medullary astrocytomas, two-stage excision may be envisaged [103].

In malignant astrocytomas, the appearance is suggestive due to the absence of a cleavage plane, with obvious infiltration of the posterior cords, the presence of foci of necrosis, the hemorrhagic character, consistency and color, which vary greatly from one tumoral focus to another, the tumour sometimes comes easily to aspiration complete resection is impossible and the aim of surgery is essentially decompression, or even simple biopsy, especially in cases where the neurological status has deteriorated [207]. Aggressive surgical resection is considered particularly in low-grade astrocytomas, as it often leads to improvement in cases in neurological transition (McCormick grade II and III), whereas its usefulness in high-grade astrocytomas is unclear. Recurrence is certain whatever the rate of excision [207].

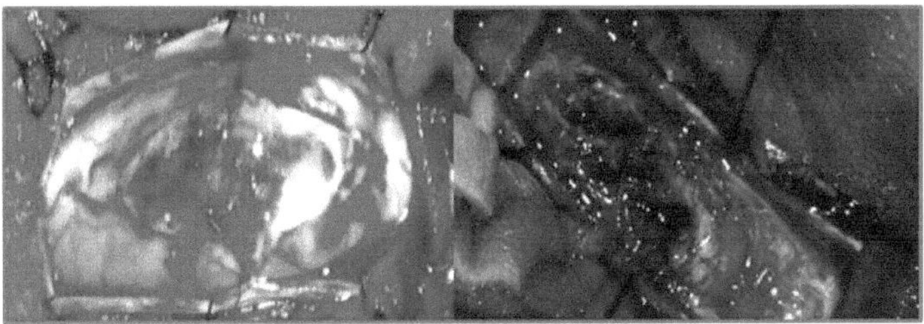

Fig. 31: Operative view of an infiltrating Astrocytoma II on the left and an infiltrating Astrocytoma II on the right.

2.4.2. Radiotherapy and chemotherapy

The value of radiotherapy remains uncertain due to the paucity of randomized astrocytoma series; however, it may be considered for high-grade malignancies, clinically progressive lesions and tumors for which extensive resection cannot be achieved [110-111-114-181].

Chemotherapy may be considered for patients with disease progression after radiotherapy, but few reports in the literature value its impact on survival [125-251-264].

A recently published multivariate study indicates that chemotherapy confers a significant improvement in PFS in patients with infiltrating astrocytomas, and that low-grade has a better prognosis [77-179].

2.4.3. Results

Total excision is achieved in 4-70% of astrocytomas [8-15-24-116-117-125-169]. Epstein [70-71] reported a 100% excision rate in two series, one adult and the other pediatric. Fischer et al [79] reported an excellent prognosis for adult patients with low-grade astrocytomas after radical resection, with survival up to 25 years. In contrast, Minehan et al [176] reported a 10-year survival rate of 81% for pilocytic astrocytomas and only 15% for astrocytoma II; moreover, patients with anaplastic astrocytomas and glioblastomas have a poor prognosis, and most die within 1 to 2 years after surgery [17-73].

Prognostic factors in patients with astrocytoma are histological grade and duration of symptom progression prior to diagnosis [133].

For glioblastoma patients, survival is generally measured in months, and those located in the cervical medulla have the poorest prognosis.

Failure is almost always due to local tumor growth at the initial site, although the possibility of simultaneous tumor dissemination throughout the neuraxis is possible, particularly with high-grade tumors [115].

3. HEMANGIOBLASTOMAS

Hemangioblastomas are highly vascular, well-limited, histologically benign and often cystic tumors; they rank third in frequency among

IMTs. Diagnosis is now possible with MRI. Treatment is surgical, as these tumors are amenable to total excision, with low morbidity and a good prognosis in sporadic cases [9].

3.1. History

The term hemangioblastoma was introduced by Cushing and Bailey in 1928, and the first successful resection of a hemangioblastoma was reported by F. Schultze in 1912. The first major series of hemangioblastoma resections, without significant morbidity, was reported in 1967 by Guidetti [94].

Microsurgery was established as a standard for hemangioblastoma excision in 1976 by Yazargil et al [268].

3.2. Epidemiology

According to the largest series, hemangioblastoma represents 2 to 15% of IMTs and 23 to 38% of CNS hemangioblastomas. They are sporadic and isolated in 2/3 of cases, or in association with VHL disease in 1/3 of cases; conversely, 60-80% of patients with VHL disease present with CNS hemangioblastoma [9-30-49-152-203].

The average age of onset is 42.5 years, with extremes ranging from 28 to 58 years [161]; this average is less than 10 years in the case of VHL [171].

There is a male predominance with a sex ratio of 1.6 to 5.5 [161], but no predominance for Klekamp, Fischer et al [79-133]. They are predominantly located in the thoracic and cervical medulla, probably in relation to the distribution and level of embryonic precursor cells [152-193-196].

3.3. Semiology

The onset of clinical signs is generally progressive, although Gautam et al [171] reported that pregnancy was a trigger and/or aggravating factor, while sometimes childbirth improved the clinical picture. Incidental findings are common in cases of VHL. The preoperative evolutionary delay varies from 1 month to 13 years [79-i33-i6i-i7i].

With regard to revealing signs, most authors stress sensory disturbances, whether or not associated with balance disorders. These signs are directly related to the anatomical location of these tumors in the posterior cords [79-i33-i7i]. Hemangioblastomas become symptomatic when they are large or associated with severe edema and/or syrinx, or sometimes, following tumor bleeding [i6i].

Clinical signs may be directly related to the tumour and/or syrinx and/or oedema, and Mandigo et col [i6i] reported patients complaining of torticollis and neurological signs in the upper limbs, despite the lesion being of thoracic location. This is due to the frequent association of haemangioblastomas with oedema and/or syringomyelia at a distance from the tumour.

In the literature, Spetzler et al [233] reported 12 cases of hemorrhage, 10 cases of subarachnoid hemorrhage and 2 cases of intramedullary hematoma. In the latter cases, the clinical picture was extremely severe (paraplegia), with no improvement after excision.

Since the advent of MRI, the majority of hemangioblastoma patients present for surgery in good functional condition (89.47 to 100% in functional grade II and III) [79-i6i].

3.4. Imaging

MRI easily establishes the diagnosis of hemangioblastoma, which is usually hyposignal to isosignal on Ti weighted sequences and isosignal or hypersignal on T2 weighted sequences. Gadolinium uptake on Ti is constant, very intense, homogeneous and total, perfectly delineating the tumor nodule.

Edema and/or peritumoral syringomyelia are well demonstrated on T2 or flair. Large lesions can be visualized without contrast medium, but small lesions are often isointense and therefore difficult to differentiate from the spinal cord, requiring gadolinium injection, which gives evocative T1-weighted images (Fig.25).

The majority of hemangioblastomas are located in the cervical and thoracic medulla [9-79-171]. Certain specific signs can help differentiate them from other tumors and vascular malformations. Hemangioblastoma usually shows homogeneous contrast with an extensive syrinx; spinal cord enlargement distant from the tumor unrelated to the syrinx is specific to hemangioblastoma. To differentiate it from arteriovenous fistulas, the latter rarely show well-limited enhancement and are typically heterogeneous without injection. Multiple hemangioblastomas have been reported only in patients with VHL disease [9-241]. Asymptomatic small hemangioblastomas may be observed in relatives of patients with VHL disease.

Patients with hemangioblastoma should benefit from contrast-enhanced MRI imaging of the entire central nervous system to exclude multiple lesions [161].

Although hemangioblastoma is a highly vascular tumor, MRI rarely reveals intramedullary or subarachnoid bleeding [233].

According to Baker's report presented at the 1999 meeting of the American Society of Neuro-radiology, 66% of spinal hemangioblastomas are straddling (intra-extramedullary, with the intramedullary portion varying in size), 25% are completely intramedullary and 8% are intradural extramedullary; 55% of hemangioblastomas have an associated cyst or syrinx and 23% of patients have the cord swollen away from the nodule and unrelated to the syrinx [161].

Pre-operative arteriography is not essential, but can help define the vascular anatomy of giant hemangioblastomas, and selective embolization remains a rare indication [42].

3.5. Histology

Macroscopically, hemangioblastomas are well-circumscribed red-orange lesions with a well-developed capsule. Their posterior location means they are sometimes hidden by posterior roots and medullary and/or radiculo-medullary blood vessels.

Microscopically (Fig. 26), hemangioblastomas are composed of a dense vascular plexus surrounded by neoplastic stromal cells. Hemangioblastomas associated with VHL disease are usually seen in young adults; and VHL disease appears to have an embryological origin derived from the mesoderm, which has the capacity to form blood and endothelial cells [196].

Hemangioblastomas, whether isolated or as part of VHL, are histologically identical, benign, richly vascularized and amenable to total excision.

Regarding the mechanism of syrinx formation, Lonser et al [152] reported a series of 22 CNS hemangioblastomas in 16 patients with VHL disease, documented with MRI. All tumors developed progressively, initially with peritumoral edema, followed by cyst formation over an average of 130 months. Vascular endothelial growth factor (VEGF) levels in the sample of tumors with syrinx at the time of resection were found to be elevated; thus cyst formation appears to be the result of increased vascular permeability of the tumor secondary to increased elevation of VEGF levels. The increased flow of interstitial fluid progressively overwhelms the absorptive capacity of the medullary tissue, and the pathological process evolves from peritumoral edema to cystic cavities, the clinical implication of which is that resection and/or fenestration of the cystic wall alone is useless; in this perspective, only complete removal of the tumor will be followed by disappearance of the cyst and/or syrinx [196].

In molecular biology, Vortmeyer and Stebbins [243-258] found a loss of heterozygosity at the VHL gene locus in stromal cells involved in the pathogenesis of hemangioblastoma.

The VHL tumor suppressor protein is known to inhibit transcriptional elongation through interaction with the Elongin protein [243]. In addition, the VHL protein also suppresses VEGF [89]. Loss of VHL protein function leads to VEGF overexpression, followed by angiogenesis [258].

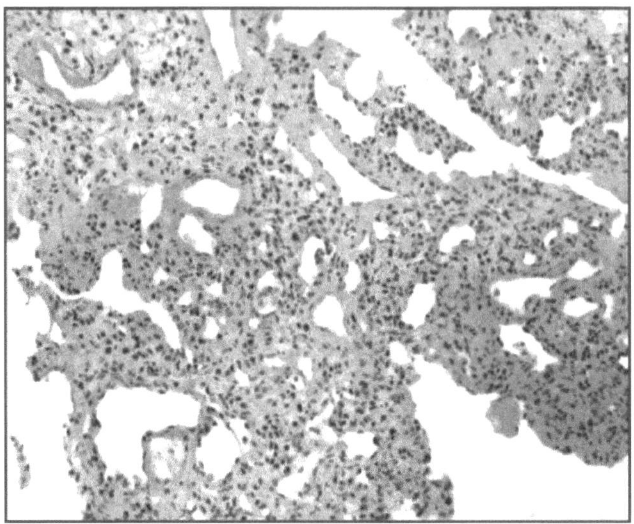

Fig. 32: Histopathology of hemangioblastoma. [212].

3.6. Treatments

Treatment of hemangioblastomas, whose technique differs from that of IMT remnants, is exclusively surgical

3.6.1. Surgical technique

The microsurgical technique has benefited greatly from the experience of certain pioneers, and the posterior approach remains by far the most widely used [196-268]. The aim of the surgical approach is to provide sufficient exposure for safe, if possible monobloc removal of the tumour.

The techniques and principles of hemangioblastoma resection (Fig. 27) differ from those used for glioma resection. Indeed, almost all glial tumors are completely intramedullary and are surgically exposed by myelotomy; whereas hemangioblastomas are considered more as juxtamedullary tumors, as they originate from the pie-mother in the vast majority of cases. This superficial situation provides the fundamental basis for surgical strategy.

Circumferential dissection of the pial attachment at the tumor/mammary interface devascularizes the tumor and provides the exposure and mobility needed to safely access and remove the intramedullary component, dissecting it from adjacent nerve structures.

Once the dura has been opened, microscopic inspection of the spinal cord allows the surface components of the tumor to be identified. Most hemangioblastomas are located on the dorsal or dorsolateral surface of the spinal cord and are easily accessible.

The superficial tumor can be recognized by its sunset-orange appearance. Large drainage veins on the dorsal and dorsolateral surface of the spinal cord are typical, and may partially or completely block visual access to the pial surface of the tumor.

The tumor may be very small and superficially located, or it may present a large exophytic component (snow cone tumor), or a very small superficial component concealing a large underlying intramedullary extension (iceberg tumor). There is also great variability in the caliber and number of superficial drainage veins. Drainage veins that block vision are systematically mobilized, coagulated and cut. More often than not, one or two large polar drainage veins are kept intact until the end of tumor resection, to avoid congestion. Dorso-lateral tumors usually involving the DREZ are covered, in part, by dorsal rootlets; these are usually mobilized and cut for at least one level to facilitate tumor removal. Once the interface between the pie-mother and the tumor has been identified, it is dissected all around. On its outer surface, an epipial arachnoid matrix is loosely attached to the pie-mother.

Unlike the brainstem, the medullary pietis is a robust membrane of longitudinally oriented fibers. Hemangioblastoma with little or no intramedullary extension is easily extirpated after detaching the circumferential margin of the tumor from the surrounding normal medulla oblongata; however, hemangioblastoma with a larger intramedullary component requires gentle traction on the tumor with either tumor forceps or a traction wire through the diseased medulla oblongata, and gradual removal of the tumor by irrigating coagulation of the tumor surface.

In whole hemangioblastomas or those with a very large intramedullary component, particularly those associated with a relatively small pial surface, a longer myelotomy is required to reveal both poles of the tumor.

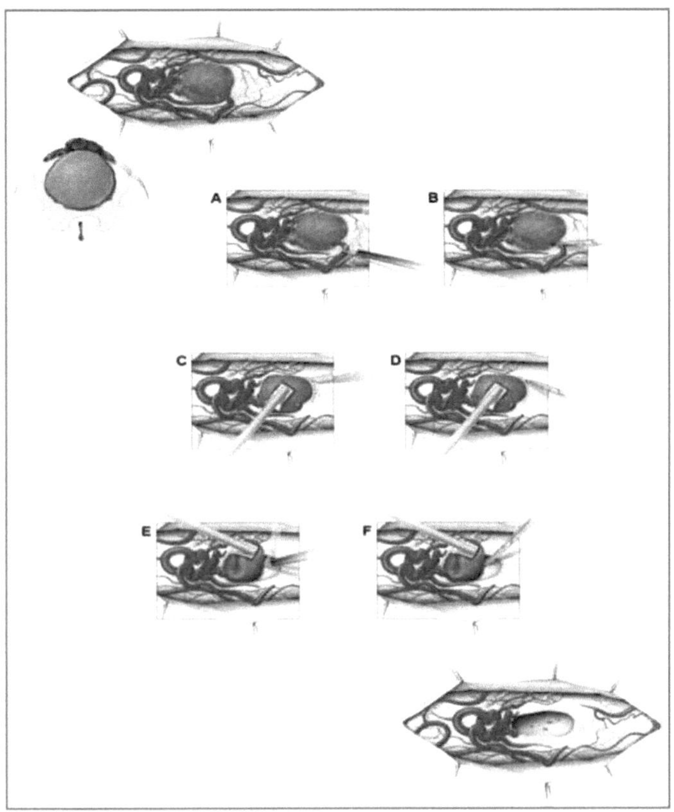

Fig. 33: Microsurgical excision technique for hemangioblastoma (**A**) (**B**): Coagulation and section of feeder vessels. **(C) (D)**: Incision of the piebrae at the edge of the tumour. **(E and F)**: Tumor dissection, the caudal pole of the IMH is lifted to expose the deep surface of the IMH, coagulation and section of the underlying vessels, and total monobloc resection. [152].

The intramedullary portion of these tumors generally presents a cleavage plane that is easily dissected, due to the frequent presence of syringomyelia. The vast majority of arterial and venous drainage in these tumors is superficial to the pie-mother. Very few feeder vessels or drainage veins are encountered during deep dissection. Bipolar coagulation of the tumour surface can reduce tumour volume and facilitate dissection, due to the fragility of the vascular stroma in hemangioblastoma [53-203-253].

Debulking and morcellation may be necessary in some cases for deep access (anterior hemangioblastoma), but these maneuvers can be perilous because of the rich vascularity. The use of videography is an adjuvant tool to ensure complete exeresis, particularly in cases of recurrence or residual hemangioblastoma [253].

In cystic forms, it is sufficient to open the cyst and remove the tumour. In the case of multiple hemangioblastomas, it is reasonable to operate only on those that are symptomatic [79-133] and, above all, to be able to treat the entire VHL disease.

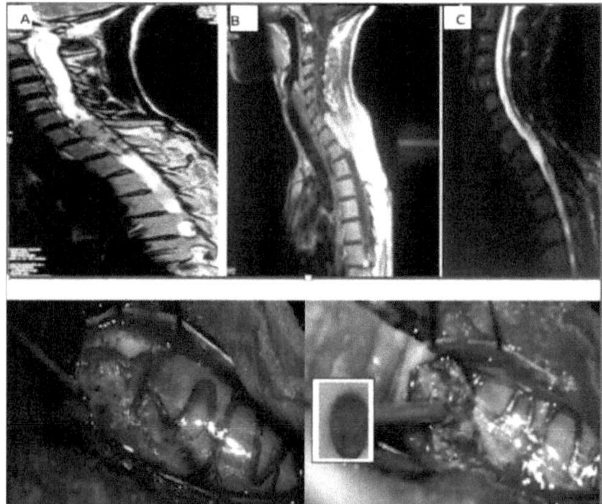

Fig. 34: Top sagittal MRI of a cervico-dorsal hemangioblastoma: A: T2: before surgery. B: T1 gado: after unsuccessful 1ere surgery (mistaken for ependymoma; error of assessment in absence of T1 gado in first stage) and C: T2 resected in its entirety after 2^{éme} surgery with resorption of syrinxes. Bottom: operative view of an exeresis.

3.6.2. Results

Preoperative neurological status and association with VHL disease are two determining factors for postoperative outcome. Thus, Van Velthoven et al [253] reported a series of 28 patients with hemangioblastomas, 64% of whom were associated with VHL disease. Excision was complete in all cases, with improvement in 28.6% and stabilization in 71.4% of patients.

Klekamp et al [133] report a total excision rate of over 90% with no permanent postoperative morbidity. Mandigo et al [161] in a series of 15 cases achieved total excision in all cases, with only two sensory aggravations recovering at 6 and 12 months postoperatively.

Recurrence, when it occurs, is certainly the consequence of incomplete resection, but other factors may have an indirect involvement, such as younger age and the presence of VHL disease.

According to Conway et al [49], recurrence occurs in around 20% of CNS hemangioblastomas.

4. CAVERNOMAS

Cavernomas are vascular malformations, angiographically occult, well circumscribed and increasingly seen in pauci- symptomatic patients since the advent of MRI [60-61].

4.1. Epidemiology

Cavernomas are considered rare, accounting for 5% of all TIMs and 5% of all CNS cavenomas [51-156].

The mean age of onset was 42 years, with no gender predominance

[93]. Nine percent of patients had a borderline family member with at least one cavernoma, and 27% of cavernomas are associated with intracranial cavernomas, with at least 45% of these cases having a family history of CNS cavernoma [20-

118-130-143].

4.2. **History and clinical presentation**

The onset of clinical signs is variable. Cavernomas tend to present with recurrent neurological signs in 16% of cases, due to repeated haemorrhage, with years separating two symptomatic phases [93-224-270]. Other patients present with slow, progressive deterioration in 54% of cases, due to asymptomatic minimal bleeding responsible over time for increased gliosis and hence spinal cord dysfunction, or in a brutal mode secondary to major bleeding in 34% of cases [33-60-192]. The acute mode is more frequently seen in children than in adults [62].

Whatever the case, changes in the lesion and/or adjacent tissue such as hyalinization, wall thickening, gliosis, changes in the microcirculation, partial thrombosis and microhemorrhages or intramedullary hematomas are the mechanisms responsible for the patterns of installation.

Diagnostic delay varies from 0 to 30 months, with an average of 7 months, and the majority of patients present in good functional condition, in McCormick grades I and II; the remainder, in grade IV, are directly related to a sudden onset secondary to major bleeding [60].

A high-quality high-field magnetic device is essential for diagnosing cavernomas, whose average size is 1cm [156].

The MRI image of the cavernoma is not pathognomonic, but is highly suggestive, appearing as a heterogeneous central zone, a mixture of predominant hypersignal (corresponding to methemoglobin testifying to recent bleeding) and hyposignal (fibrosis-calcifications), and a hypointense peripheral zone forming a ring (corresponding to hemosiderin, the final degradation product of hemoglobin) (Fig. 28). Multi-planar slices help to determine the best indications for surgery. Medullary arteriography is normal, due to the low-pressure flow that characterizes these angiographically occult lesions.

Multiple forms have been described, particularly in familial forms.

4.4. Histology

Macroscopically, it is a reddish mass, sub-centimetric in diameter, with a poly-lobed surface and a clear boundary with the adjacent medullary parenchyma, although it generally lacks a capsule. Its arterial vascularization is ensured by arterioles visible only under the microscope.

Cavernomas are histologically identical to their intracranial counterparts (Fig. 29). They are made up of juxtaposed communicating cavities, blood-filled caverns separated by collagenous tissue lined with endothelium. The surrounding nervous tissue may be the site of gliosis or remodelling. Blood circulates in the cavities under low pressure, which explains the frequency of intracavitary thrombosis, which in turn progresses to fibrosis and calcification. The pericavernomatous medullary tissue has a characteristic operative appearance; it is greenish-yellow, testifying to the existence of long-standing iterative microhemorrhagic phenomena. After a period of quiescence, the spontaneous evolution of these lesions may be marked by acute haemorrhage (due to rupture of a surface cavern).

4.5. Treatment and results

Surgery should be considered for cavernomas of incidental and/or pauci-symptomatic discovery, as soon as the diagnosis is made, partly because of the risk of spontaneous bleeding, and partly because of the low morbidity of surgery.

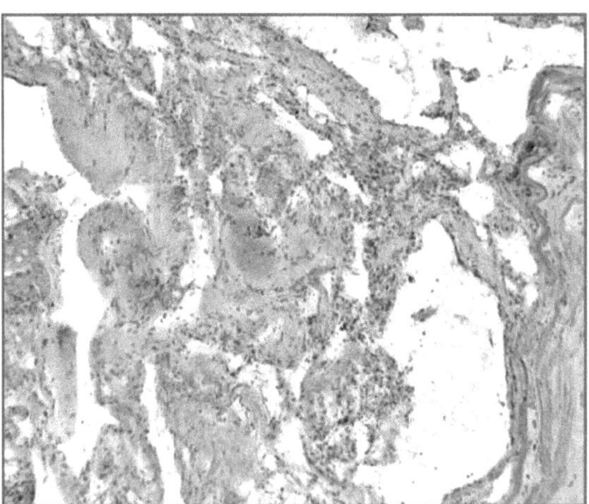

Fig. 35: Histopathology of Cavernoma[212].

4.5.1. Surgery

Surgery is the exclusive treatment. However, the problem of surgical indications arises (Fig.30) due to the large number of asymptomatic cavernomas discovered as part of extension work-ups and/or screening. For the latter, Cantore et al [33] recommend abstention and regular monitoring of these patients. Ojemann et al [192] suggest immediate surgery, provided they are posterior in location (favorable position for resection). The risk of spontaneous bleeding is approximately 1.6

% per patient/year [32]. Sandalcioglu et al [224] found a higher bleeding rate of 4.5% per patient/year and a rebleeding rate of 66% per patient/year.

Cervical cavernomas are considered particularly susceptible to clinical worsening [32]. In view of the enormous serious consequence of intramedullary hemorrhage and the low surgical morbidity, abstention is justified only for deep asymptomatic cavernomas far from the pie-me according to Ojemann [192].

The surgical technique obeys the same rules of excision applied to other TIMs. The surgeon must carefully analyze the preoperative MRI in relation to the superficial subpial location of cavernomas, since according to Vishteh et al [255], there is a false-positive rate of 17.6% (superficial location) when the lesion is deeper intraoperatively. The approach to these lesions involves laminectomy or hemilaminectomy. The anterior approach by partial corporectomy to tackle anterior cervical cavernomas remains the exception [187].

Exophytic lesions, staining or swelling of the medullary surface can guide myelotomy. Deep lesions can be approached via median myelotomy or DREZ, guided by real-time intraoperative ultrasound, the latter also helping to perfect total excision. Once the cavernoma has been reached, the feeding arteries and draining veins are coagulated and cut; small cotton balls are placed between the malformation and the parenchyma in the stained hemosiderin deposit. A cleavage plane is usually present, and the lesion is removed en bloc or by morcellation. Supernumerary vascular malformations may coexist and must be resected, as they may be a source of rebleeding [156-255].

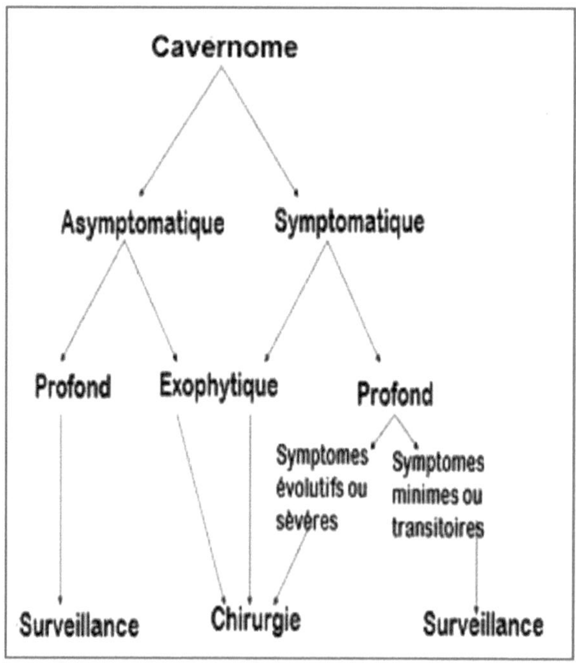

Fig. 36: Algorithm for the management of cavernomas. [93].

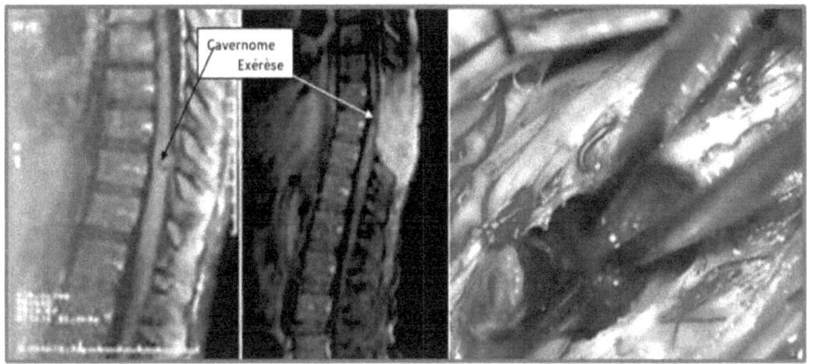

Fig. 37: Pre- and postoperative sagittal MRI and operative view of total resection

4.5.2. Results

According to Daniel, Gross et al [57-93], exeresis is total in 91% to 100% of cases, 41% to 61% of patients are improved, 27% to 50% are stable and 9% to 12% are worsened, and postoperative morbidity is of the order of 36%.

5. METASTASES

Intramedullary metastases are rare complications of systemic cancers [39]. In the SNCLF series, metastases account for 4% of IMTs, and Fischer [79] found only two cases.

The main clinical features are altered general condition and rapid progression of neurological deficit [52].

MRI is undoubtedly the most sensitive and specific examination for detecting metastases. Injection of gadolinium enables the tumour site to be distinguished from reactive oedema, helping to better plan surgery (Fig.31). MRI is also effective for identifying other neuraxial localizations and monitoring response to treatment.

The incidence of metastases is higher in patients with lung cancer, accounting for 41% of the 100 cases of metastases reported in the literature [122]. Watanabe et al [260] reported four small-cell carcinomas, one lung adenocarcinoma, one uterine carcinoma and one breast carcinoma.

According to Kalayci et al [126], primary surgical resection resulted in improvement in 77% of cases, while 23% remained unchanged. Surgery probably offered patients in good clinical condition a better outcome, but these figures do not justify broadly recommending surgery for these patients.

In Sakuma's series [220], only partial excision was performed and no neurological improvement was observed.

In conclusion, metastases are rare complications of systemic cancers. Their MRI characteristics are similar to those of brain metastases. Surgical treatment is rarely indicated, but radiotherapy is recommended.

6. THE HAMARTOMS

Hamartomas are not tumors in the strict sense, due to the absence of tumor cell proliferation, but they occupy space and exert a mass effect on the medullary tissue. In most cases, they are not completely surrounded by the medullary tissue, and have a component of extramedullary. Thus, they are classified as intramedullary only if the major component of the lesion is lodged in the spinal cord [79].

6.1. Lipomas

Non-dysraphic intramedullary lipoma is a rare tumor, accounting for less than 1% of all IMTs, mostly affecting young adults, and exceptionally children; the mean age of onset is 35 years [133]. According to Fischer and Brotchi [79], lipomas account for 6.4% of IMTs.

Lipomas increase in size over time due to the hypertrophy of lipomatous tissue that occurs whenever there are changes in the body's adipose tissue in general; in other words, lipomas can be reduced in size by following a low-fat diet and losing weight [69]; they also increase in size during corticosteroid therapy [3].

The pre-operative history tends to be longer than that of other IMT entities.

Symptomatology is dominated by pain or sphincter disorders. Computed tomography may show a hypodense intramedullary lesion, but MRI remains the examination of choice for diagnosis, showing a hypersignal image in T1-weighted sequence and hyposignal in T2-weighted sequence with no change in signal after gadolinium injection, and disappearing in fat saturation sequence (Fig. 32).

Lipomas do not present a cleavage plane and behave like an infiltrating neoplasm; consequently, complete resection of a lipoma is not recommended and decompression is the procedure of choice [65-67-131]. Several authors recommend the use of the carbon dioxide laser for their excision [170].

For Lee [148], pain may be improved, but he found no change in neurological status. For Klelamp et al [133], 2/5 of patients improved and

3 worsened with a dysesthetic syndrome, two of which were complicated by progressive myelopathy linked to a post-fixed spinal cord.

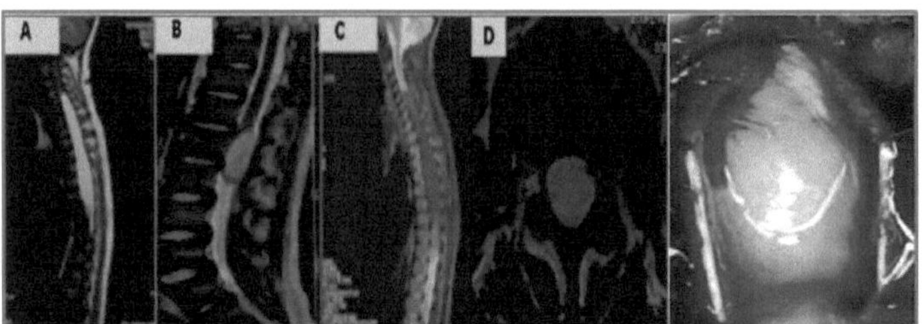

Fig. 38: Sagittal T1, T2 and axial MRI and operative view of a bipolar lipoma.

6.2. Dermoid and epidermoid cysts

Dermoid and epidermoid cysts are benign, slow-growing tumoral formations, almost always congenital in origin, resulting from aberrant inclusion of ectodermal elements during neural tube closure between $3^{\text{ème}}$ and $5^{\text{ème}}$ weeks of embryonic development; however, if iatrogenic, they are often extramedullary.

The cysts contain secretory cells responsible for its expansion. In the SNCLF series [79], they account for 2.9% of IMDs, with a mean age at diagnosis of 32 years.

The history is much shorter than for lipomas. On average, it lasts 51 months [133]. Clinical symptomatology is not pathognomonic, but acute pictures have been described and are linked to aseptic meningitis [226] or abscess formation [45].

MRI, as for all IMT, is the key examination for the diagnosis of dermoid and epidermoid cysts, whose appearance is reminiscent of intracranial localizations, with hypersignal in both sequences for dermoid cysts and iso/hyposignal in T1 and hypersignal in T2 for epidermoid cysts, although mixed signals have been reported (Fig.33) [55-79].

These lesions are treated surgically, with the aim of complete removal. Opening the capsule allows easy removal of the soft cystic contents, thus saving space and reducing any inadvertent mobilization of adjacent nerve structures. Unlike intracranial procedures, cleavage between the capsule and the medulla is often difficult due to adhesions. In such cases, it may be wise to settle for an incomplete excision, given the functional risks involved, especially as recurrence is low and will occur as slowly as the clinical history [4-55-79].

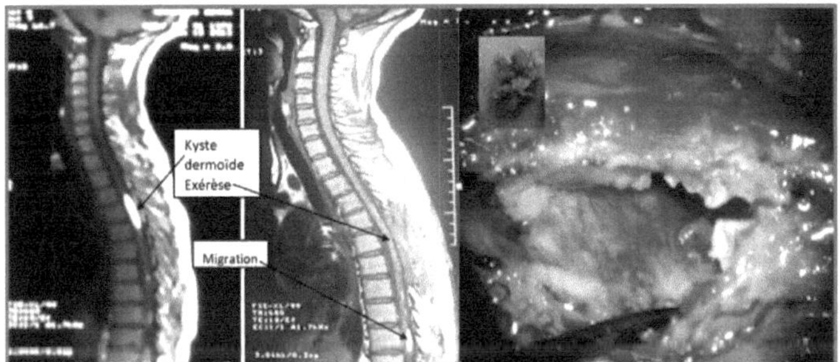

Fig. 40: Pre- and postoperative MRI and operative view of a dermoid cyst with leakage of lipid droplets into the ependymal canal after excision. Right: operative view.

7. MELANOCYTOMAS

Primary melanoma is a rare tumor, first reported in 1972 by Limas and Tio, and since then around 100 cases have been reported in the CNS (brain and spinal cord) [5]. It occurs predominantly in middle-aged adults, with no gender predominance. Diagnosis takes an average of one year. Symptoms are mainly of lower limb deficits, in direct relation to the preferred thoracic site. Spinal pain is present in 60-85% of cases. Cerebrospinal fluid is often pathological, sometimes xanthochromic and exceptionally black. MRI is of particular interest due to the paramagnetic behavior of melanin contained in melanocytes. It shows a relative hypersignal in T1 weighting and proton density, and a hyposignal in T2 weighting (Fig. 34). In the presence of an intramedullary lesion with paramagnetic signal, several diagnostic hypotheses are possible, in particular a primary or secondary melanoma, a lipoma or a hemorrhagic lesion.

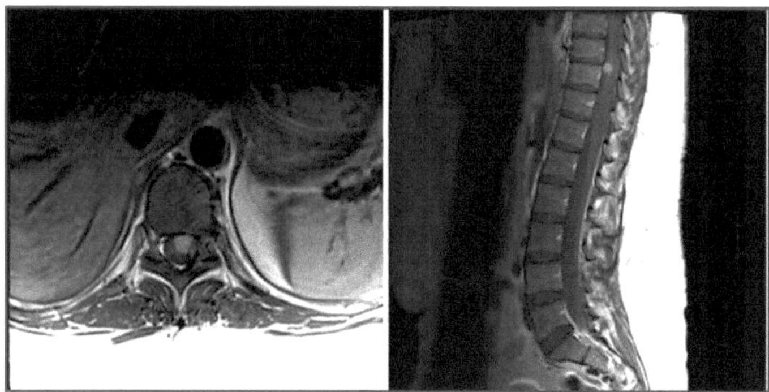

Fig. 41: T1 MRI with gadolinium: T9-T10 intramedullary melanocytoma, homogeneously enhanced.

Intramedullary melanocytoma is considered primitive when no other melanocytoma is found outside the central nervous system. Its location is usually middle or lower thoracic.

Treatment is not codified, but often combines surgery and radiotherapy. MRI scans should be performed at a distance to check for local recurrence or prognostic leptomeningeal metastases [14-88-158-248].

8. EPENDYMOGLIAL CYSTS

Formerly called terminal ventricles because of their frequency in the conus medullaris, they are now ubiquitous and are essential in adulthood [46-213].

MRI can easily be used to diagnose, evaluate and differentiate cysts, which are well-limited, usually anterior and eccentric to the canal, with a signal identical to the LCS (Fig.35However, the diagnostic criteria for syringomyelia are based essentially on the shape and size of the cyst, which leads to symmetrical bipolar expansion without septa of the medulla, whereas syringomyelia tends to taper at both ends [238].

Most authors consider that the ependymoglial cyst is the consequence of a proliferation of ectopic ependymal cells [82].

Pathologically, the ependymal cyst is characterized by a lining of epithelium overlying fibrous tissue without basement membrane interposition. The cyst content is a clear fluid reminiscent of CSF, but may also be thick and protein-rich [82].

Treatment is exclusively surgical in symptomatic cases, and consists of drainage of the cyst into the subarachnoid space, with this communication being maintained either by eversion of the cystic border or sometimes by interposition of a shunt. The earlier the patient is operated on, the better the results [219].

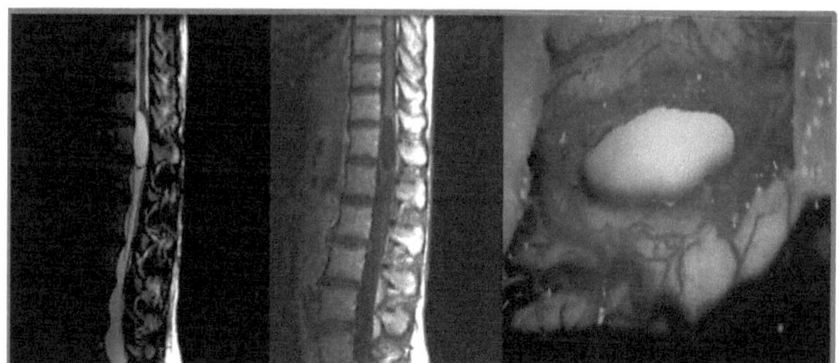

Fig.42: Sagittal MRI T2, T1 and operative view of an ependymo-glial cyst of the terminal cone. Right: operative view.

9. OTHER TIM

Meningiomas, schwannomas, primary lymphomas, metastases of malignant brain tumors, sarcoidosis and other glial entities are rare [79128-129-133-175-189].

VII. CONCLUSION

IMTs are rare lesions that require particular clinical lucidity and a rapid diagnostic approach, as only an early diagnosis at a preserved functional stage can guarantee a favorable post-operative outcome.

So, while it's vital to have good clinicians for a better diagnostic approach and experienced neurosurgeons, it's even more important to provide easy access to MRI imaging, which should be generalized in public hospitals.

The rarity of these lesions makes the creation of a specialized center for spinal cord surgery an absolute priority, and may be considered the only means within our reach at the present time, capable of optimizing the results of these lesions thanks to targeted recruitment and therefore better management.

The importance of early diagnosis must be clearly emphasized, in order to intervene without delay and achieve total excision; this objective seems to be achievable for patients in good functional condition and with benign or low-grade malignant IMT, but without putting patients at major functional risk.

Intraoperative neurophysiological monitoring is a key tool for optimizing the quality of exeresis and minimizing operative risks; however, other technical means such as CUSA and intraoperative ultrasound appear to be an important asset in the surgical arsenal, improving above all the surgeon's comfort.

We hope that this initiative will pave the way for further efforts to better analyze and manage these lesions.

The prognosis and outcome of long-term management of IMT

is favorable, particularly for benign IMT, which accounts for the majority of these lesions, provided they are ready for total exeresis. The role and benefits of adjuvant therapy, i.e. radiation and chemotherapy, are not yet well established.

BIBLIOGRAPHY

1. Abdel-Wahab M, Corn B, Wolfson A: Prognostic factors and survival in patients with spinal cord gliomas after radiation therapy. Am J Clin Oncol 1999, 22: 344-5.

2. Aghakhani N, David P, Parker F: Intramedullary spinal ependymoma: analysis of a consecutive series of 82 adult cases with particular attention to patients with no preoperative neurological deficit. Neurosurgery 2008, 62: 1279-1285.

3. Agraharkar A, McGillicuddy G, Ahuja T: Growth of intramedullary lipoma in a renal transplant recipient. Transplantation 2000, 69: 1509-1511.

4. Akhaddar A, El Hassani MY, Ghadouane M: Dermoid cyst of the medullary cone revealed by chronic retention of urine. Journal of Neuroradiology 1999,26/2, p. 132.

5. Allan H, Friedman Isaac O, Karikari O: Primary intramedullary melanocytoma of the spinal cord: case report. Neurosurgery 2009, 64: E777-E778.

6. Allen JC, Aviner S, Yates AJ: Children's Cancer Group Treatment of high-grade spinal cord astrocytoma of childhood with "8-in-1" chemotherapy and radiotherapy: a pilot study of CCG-945. J Neurosurg 1998, 88: 215-220.

7. Alter M: Tumours of the spine and spinal cord. Edited by Klawans HL (editor). Amsterdam: American Elsevier: 2008, 55-61.

8. Alvisi C, Cerisoli M, Giulioni M: Intramedullary spinal gliomas: long-term results of surgical treatment.Acta Neurochir (Wien). 1984, 70: 169-179.

9. Ammerman JM, Lonser RR, Dambrosia J: Long term natural history of hemangioblastomas in patients with Von Hippel-Lindau disease: Implications for treatment. J Neurosurg 2006, 105: 248-255.

10. Anakwenze OA, Auerbach JD, Buck DW: The role of concurrent fusion to prevent spinal deformity after intramedullary spinal cord tumor excision in children. J Pediatr Orthop. 2011, Jul-Aug; 31(5): 475-9.

11. Anderson.M: tumors of the brain and spine. Springer Science+Business Media, LLC, 2007, p. 312.

12. Ardeshiri A, Chen B, Hütter BO, Oezkan N, Wanke I, Sure U, Sandalcioglu IE. Intramedullary spinal cord astrocytomas: the influence of localization and tumor extension on resectability and functional outcome. Acta Neurochir (Wien). 2013 Jul;155(7).

13. Balmaceda C: Chemotherapy for intramedullary spinal cord tumors. Neurooncol. 2000, May; 47 (3):293-307.

14. Barth A, Pizzolato GP, Berney J: Intramedullary meningeal melanocytoma. Neurosurgery. 1993, 19:188-194.

15. Bazan Cd, New PZ, Kagan-Hallet KS: MRI of radiation induced spinal cord glioma. Neuroradiology, 1990, 32:331-333.

16. Beck OJ: The use of the Nd-YAG and the CO2 laser in neurosurgery. Neurosurg Rev, 1980, 3: 261-266.

17. BenesV, Barsa P, Benes V: Prognostic factors in intramedullary astrocytomas; a literature review. Eur Spine J. 2009; 18(10):1397-1422.

18. Berhouma M, Bahri K, Houissa S: Management of intramedullary spinal cord tumors: surgical considerations and results in 45 cases. Neurosurgery 2009, 55(3):293-302.

19. Bhatoe HS, Singh P, Chaturvedi A: Nondysraphic intramedullary spinal cord lipomas: a review. Neurosurg Focus 2005, 18 (2):ECP1.

20. Bian LG, Bertalanffy H, Sun QF: Intramedullary cavernous malformations: clinical features and surgical technique via hemilaminectomy. Clin Neurol Neurosurg 2009, 111:511-517.

21. Bostrom A, Hans FJ, Reinacher PC: Intramedullary hemangioblastomas: timing of surgery, microsurgical technique and follow-up in 23 patients. Eur Spine J. 2008, Jun; 17(6):882-6.

22. Bostrom A, Von Lehe M, Hartmann W: Surgery for spinal cord ependymomas; outcome and prognostic factors. Neurosurgery. 2011, 68:302-309.

23. Bouaziz M. C. Daghfous M. S. Ladeb M. F: Childhood scoliosis revealing spinal cord tumorsur .J Orthop Surg Traumatol 2006, 16: 318-321.

24. Bouffet E, Pierre-Kahn A, Marchal J C: Prognostic factors in pediatric spinal cord astrocytoma. Cancer 1998, 83:2391-2399.

25. Boyd SG, Rothwell JC, Cowan JM: A method of monitoring function in corticospinal pathways during scoliosis surgery with a note on motor conduction velocities.
J Neurol Neurosurg Psychiatry 1986,49/3:251-7.

26. Brotchi J, Dewitte O, Levivier M: A survey of 65 tumors within the spinal cord: surgical results and the importance of preoperative magnetic resonance imaging. Neurosurgery 1991, 29:651-656.

27. Brotchi J, Fischer G: Spinal cord ependymomas. Neurosurg Focus 1998, 15; 4(5):e2.

28. Brotchi J: Intrinsic spinal cord tumor resection. Neurosurgery 2002, 50:1059-1063.

29. Brotchi J, Bruneau M, Lefranc F: Surgery of Intraspinal Cord Tumors. Clin

Neurosurg. 2006,53:209-216.

30. Browne TR, Adams RD, Roberson GH: Hemangioblastoma of the spinal cord. Review and report of five cases. Arch Neurol 1976, 33:435-441.

31. Bulsara KR, Sukhla S, Nimjee SM: History of bipolar coagulation. Neurosurg Rev 2006, 29:93-96.

32. Canavero S, Pagni CA, Duca S: Spinal intramedullary cavernous angiomas; a literature meta-analysis. Surg Neurol 1994, 41:381-388.

33. Cantore G, Delfini R, Cervoni L: Intramedullary cavernous angiomas of the spinal cord: report of six cases. Surg Neurol 1995, 43:448-451.

34. Cantore G, Ciappetta P, Santoro A: Discontinuous myelotomy; an alternative to standard myelotomy in the surgical treatment of intramedullary spinal cord tumours. Acta Neurochir (Wien) 2002, Apr; 144(4):373-6.

35. CBTRUS: http://www.cbtrus.org/reports//2007.

36. Chamberlain MC: Etoposide for recurrent spinal cord ependymoma. Neurology 2002, 23; 58(8):1310-1.

37. Chandler WF, Knake JE: Intraoperative use of ultrasound in neurosurgery. Clin Neurosurg 1983, 31: 550-563.

38. Chang UK, Choe WJ, Chung SK: Surgical outcome and prognostic factors of spinal intramedullary ependymomas in adults. J Neurooncol 2002, 57: 133-139.

39. Chason JL, Walker FB, Landers JW: Metastatic carcinoma in the central nervous system and dorsal root Ganglia a prospective autopsy study. Cancer 1963, 16: 781-787.

40. Chigasaki H, Pennybacker JB: A long follow-up study of 128 cases of intramedullary spinal cord tumours.Neurol Med Chir (Tokyo) 1968, 10: 25-66.

41. Chun H, Schmidt-Ullrich R, Wolfson A, Tercilla O: External beam radiotherapy for primary spinal cord tumors. J Neurooncol 1990, 9: 211-217.

42. Clark AJ, Lu DC, Richardson RM: Surgical technique of temporary arterial occlusion in the operative management of spinal hemangioblastomas. World Neurosurg. 2010, Jul; 74(1): 200-5.

43. Cloyd MW: Low FN: Scanning electron microscopy of the subarachnoid space in the dog. I.Spinal cord levels. J Comp Neurol 1974, 153:325-368.

44. Cohen-Gadol AA, Jacob JT, Edwards DA: Coexistence of intracranial and spinal cavernous malformations: a study of prevalence and natural history. J Neurosurg 2006, 104:376-381.

45. Cokca F, Meco O, Arasil E: An intramedullary dermoid cyst abscess due to Brucella abortus biotype 3 at T11-L2 spinal levels. Infection 1994, 22: 359-360.

46. Coleman LT, Zimmerman RA, Rorke LB: Ventriculus terminalis of the conus medullaris: MR findings in children.AJNR Am J Neuroradiol 1995, 16:1421-1426.

47. Colnat-Coulbois S, Klein O, Braun M: Management of Intramedullary Cystic Pilocytic Astrocytoma With Rhenium-186 Intracavitary Irradiation: Case Report. Neurosurgery 2010, 66:E1023-E1024.

48. Constantini S, Miller DC, Allen JC: Radical excision of intramedullary spinal cord tumors: surgical morbidity and long term follow-up evaluation in 164 children and young adults. JNeurosurg 2000, 93:183-193.

49. Conway JE, Chou D, Clatterbuck R: Hemangioblastomas of the central nervous system in von Hippel-Lindau syndrome and sporadic disease. Neurosurgery 2001, 48:55-63.

50. Cooper PR: Outcome after operative treatment of intramedullary spinal cord tumors in adults: intermediate and long-term results in 51 patients. Neurosurg 1989, 25: 855-859.

51. Cosgrove GR, Bertrand G, Fontaine S: Cavernous angiomas of the spinal cord. JNeurosurg 1988, .68:31-36.

52. Costigan DA, Winkelman MD: Intramedullary spinal cord metastasis. A clinicopathological study of 13 cases. J Neurosurg 1985, 62:227-233.

53. Cristante L, Herrmann HD: Surgical management of intramedullary hemangioblastoma of the spinal cord. Acta Neurochir (Wien) 1999, 141:333-340.

54. Crowley RW, Sherman JH, Le BH, Jane JA Sr: intramedullary spinal cord metastasis from bladder carcinoma: case report Neurosurg 2008, 63:E611-E612.

55. Cupta S, Gupta RK, Gujral RB: Signal intensity patterns in intraspinal dermoids and epidermoids on MR imaging .Clinical Radiology 1993, 48/6,405-413.

56. Damadian R: Tumor detection by nuclear magnetic resonance. Science 1971, 171:1151-1153.

57. Daniel C. Lu, Michael T: Clinical presentation and surgical management of intramedullary spinal cord cavernous malformations Neurosurg Focus 2010, 29 (3):E12.

58. Daniel T, Nagasawa, B.A, Zachary A: Complications associated with the treatment for spinal ependymomas Neurosurg Focus 2011, 31 (4):E13.

59. Deletis V: Intraoperative neurophysiology and methodologies used to monitor the functional integrity of the motor system. In: Deletis V, Shils J (eds)

Neurophysiology in neurosurgery: a modern intraoperative approach. Academic, San Diego, 2002: 25-50.

60. Deutsch H, Jallo GI, Epstein F: Spinal intramedullar cavernoma: clinical presentation and surgical outcome. J Neurosurg 2000, 93 (1 Suppl):65-70.

61. Deutsch H: Pain outcomes after surgery in patients with intramedullary spinal cord cavernous malformations. Neurosurgery Focus, 2010, Sep; (3) :E15.

62. DeutschH, Shrivistava R, Epstein F: Pediatric intramedullary spinal cavernous malformations. Spine 2001, 26:E427-E431.

63. Djindjian R: Vascular malformations. In: Shapiro R (ed) Myelography, 4th edn. Year Book Medical Publishers, Chicago, 1984.

64. Dow G, Biggs N, Evans G: Spinal tumors in neurofibromatosis type 2. Is emerging knowledge of genotype predictive of natural history? J Neurosurg Spine 2005, 2:574-579.

65. Dyck P: Intramedullary lipoma. Diagnosis and treatment. Spine 1992, 17:979-981.

66. Ebert C, Von Haken M, Meyer-Puttlitz B: Molecular genetic analysis of ependymal tumors. NF2 mutations and chromosome 22q loss occur preferentially in intramedullary spinal ependymomas. Am J Pathol. 1999, Aug; 155(2):627-32.

67. El Khamlichi A, El Ouahabi A, Amrani F, Agdach R, Bellakhdar F: Intramedullary lipoma. A propos de 3 cas. Neurochirurgie. 1989; 35(6):366-70.

68. El Negamy E, Sedgwick EM: Delayed cervical somatosensory potentials in cervical spondylosis. J Neurol Neurosurg Psychiatry 1979, 42:238-241.

69. Endoh M, Iwasaki Y, Koyanagi I· Spontaneous shrinkage of lumbosacral lipoma in conjunction with a general decrease in body fat: case report. Neurosurgery 1998, 43/1:150-1.

70. Epstein F, Epstein N: Surgical treatment of spinal cord astrocytomas of childhood. A series of 19 patients. J Neurosurg 1982, 57:685-689.

71. Epstein F: Spinal cord astrocytomas of childhood. Adv Tech Stand Neurosurg 1986, 13:135-169.

72. Epstein FJ, Farmer JP, Freed D: Adult intramedullary spinal cord ependymomas: the results of surgery in 38 patients. J Neurosurg 1993, 79:204-209.

73. Epstein FJ, Farmer JP, Freed D: Adult intramedullary astrocytomas of the spinal cord. J Neurosurg 1992, 77: 355-359.

74. Epstein FJ, Farmer JP, Schneider SJ: Intraoperative ultrasonography an important surgical adjunct for intramedullary tumors. J Neurosurg 1991, 74/5:729-33.

75. Eroes CA, Zausinger S, Kreth FW: Intramedullary low grade astrocytoma and ependymoma. Surgical results and predicting factors for clinical outcome. Acta Neurochir (Wien). Apr; 152 (4):611-8.

76. Fakhrai N, Neophytou P, Dieckmann K, Nemeth A: Recurrent spinal ependymoma showing partial remission under Imatimib. Acta Neurochir (Wien). 2004, Nov; 146(11):1255-8.

77. Fakhreddine MH, Mahajan A, Penas-Prado M: Treatement, prognostic factors, and outcomes in spinal cord astrocytomas. Neuro-Oncology. 2013 Apr; 15(4):406-12.

78. Ferrante L, Mastronardi L, Celli P, Lunardi P, Acqui M: Intramedullary spinal cord ependymomas a study of 45 cases with long-term follow-up. Acta Neurochir (Wien). 1992, 119:74-79.

79. Fischer G, Brotchi J: Intramedullary tumors. Report of the Societé Francaise de Neurochirurgie. 45eme congres annuel. Angers, June 15- 12-1994. Neurochirurgie. 1994, 40 Suppl 1: 1-108.

80. Flamm ES, Ransohoff J, Wuchinich D: Preliminary experience with ultrasonic aspiration in neurosurgery. Neurosurgery. 1978, 2:240-245.

81. Forster MT, Marquardt G, Seifert V, Szelényi A: Spinal Cord Tumor SurgeryImportance of Continuous Intraoperative Neurophysiological Monitoring After Tumor Resection. Spine. Vol 37, Number 16, pp E1001-E1008.

82. FortunaA, Mercuri S: Intradural spinal cysts. ActaNeurochir (Wien). 1983, 68:289314.

83. Garcés-Ambrossi GL, McGirt MJ, Mehta VA, Sciubba DM: Factors associated with progression free survival and longterm neurological outcome after resection of intramedullary spinal cord tumors: analysis of 101 consecutive cases. J Neurosurg Spine. 2009, Nov; 11(5):591-9.

84. Garcia DM: Primary spinal cord tumors treated with surgery and postoperative irradiation. Int J Radiat Oncol Biol Phys. 1985, 11/11:1933-1939.

85. Gavin Quigley D, Farooqi N, Pigott TJ: Outcome predictors in the management of spinal cord ependymoma. Eur Spine J. 2007, 16(3):399-404.

86. Glasker S, Shah MJ, Hippchen B, Neumann HP, van Velthoven V: Doppler-sonographically guided resection of central nervous system hemangioblastomas. Neurosurgery. 2011. Jun; 68(2 Suppl Operative):267-75.

87. Glasker S, Van Velthoven V: Risk of hemorrhage in hemangioblastomas of the central nervous system. Neurosurgery. 2005, 57:71-76.

88. Glick R, Baker C, Husain S: Primary melanocytomas of the spinal cord: a report of seven cases. Clin Neuropathol. 1997, 16:127-132.

89. Gnarra JR, Zhou S, Merrill MJ: Post-transcriptional regulation of vascular endothelial growth factor mRNA by the product of the VHL tumor suppressor gene. Proc Natl Acad Sci U S A. 1996, 93:10589-10594.

90. Goh KY, Velasquez L, Epstein FJ: Pediatric intramedullary spinal cord tumors: is surgery alone enough? Pediatr Neurosurg. 1997, 27:34-39.

91. Greenwood J Jr: Intramedullary tumors of spinal cord. A follow- up study after total surgical removal. J Neurosurg. 1963, 20:665-668.

92. Gregory D. Cramer: basic and clinical anatomy of the spine, spinal cord and ans, by Mosby6ed:1995.63-68.

93. Gross BA, Du R, Popp AJ, Day AL: Intramedullary spinal cord cavernous malformations. Neurosurg Focus. 2010, Sep;29(3):E14.

94. Guidetti B, Fortuna A: Surgical treatment of intramedullary hemangioblastoma of the spinal cord. Report of six cases. J Neurosurg. 1967, 27:530-540.

95. Guidetti B, Mercuri B, Vagnozzi R: Long-term results of the surgical treatment of 129 intramedullary spinal gliomas. J Neurosurg. 1981, 54:323-330.

96. Halvorsen CM, Kolstad F, Hald J: Long-term Outcome After Resection of Intraspinal Ependymomas: Report of 86 Consecutive Cases. Neurosurgery. 2010, 67:1622-1631.

97. Hanbali F, Fourney DR, Marmor E: Spinal cord ependymoma radical surgical resection and outcome. Neurosurgery. 2002, 51:1162-1172.

98. Hara Y, Tamaki N, Nakamura M, Nagashima T, Yamashita H, Takaishi Y: A new technique for intraoperative visual monitoring during spinal surgery: angiofiber and endoscopic ultrasonography. J Clin Neurosci. 2001, Jul; 8(4):347-50.

99. Harrop JS, Ganju A, Groff M, Bilsky M: Primary intramedullary tumors of the spinal cord. Spine (Phila Pa 1976). 2009, Oct 15; 34(22 Suppl):S69-77.

100. Hausmann ON, Kirsch EC, Tolnay M, Gratzl O: Intramedullary spinal cord tumours: a clinical outcome and radiological follow-up study. Swiss Med Wkly. 131:582-587, 2001.

101. Henson JW: Spinal cord gliomas. Current Opinion in Neurology. 2001, 14:679-682.

102. Herrmann HD, Neuss M, Winkler D: intramedullary spinal cord tumors resected with CO2 Laser Microsurgical techniques: recent experience in fifteen patient. Neurosurgery. 1988, 22(3):518-22.

103. Hida K, Iwasaki Y, Seki T: tow stage operation for resection of spinal cord astrocytoma; technical case report of thre Cases. Neurosurgery. 2006, 58[ONS Suppl 2]: ONS-373-ONS-374.

104. Holland EC: Gliomagenesis: genetic alterations and mouse models. Nat Rev Genet. 2001, 2:120-129.

105. Holland EC: Progenitor cells and glioma formation. Curr Opin Neurol. 2001,14:683-688.

106. HorwitzNH: Charles A. Elsberg (1871-1948). Neurosurgery. 1997, 40:1315-1319.

107. Hoshimaru M, Koyama T, Hashimoto N: Results of microsurgical treatment for intramedullary spinal cord ependymomas: analysis of 36 cases. Neurosurgery. 1999, 44:264-269.

108. Houten JK, Cooper PR: Spinal cord astrocytomas: presentation, management and outcome. J Neurooncol. 2000, 47:219-224.

109. Houten JK, Weiner HL: Pediatric intramedullary spinal cord tumors: special considerations. JNeurooncol. 2000, 47:225-230.

110. Huddart R, Traish D, Ashley S, Moore A, Brada M: Management of spinal astrocytoma with conservative surgery and radiotherapy. Br J Neurosurg. 1993, 7:473-481.

111. Hulshof MC, Menten J, Dito JJ, Dreissen JJR, Van den Bergh R, Gonzalez D: Treatment results in primary intraspinal gliomas. Radiat Oncol 29: 294-300, 1993

112. Hurth.M, David.P: les astrocytomes intramédullaires: conduite à tenir. La Lettre du Neurologue. 2002,6/ 5,165-167.

113. Innocenzi G, Raco A, Cantore G: Intramedullary astrocytomas and ependymomas in the pediatric age group: a retrospective study. Childs Nerv Syst. 1996, 12:776-780.

114. Isaacson SR: Radiation therapy and the management of intramedullary spinal cord tumors. JNeurooncol. 2000, 47(3):231-8.

115. Ito U, Tomita H, Yamazaki S, Takada Y, Inaba YCT: findings of leptomeningeal and periventricular dissemination of tumors. Report of four cases. Clin Neurol Neurosurg. 1986, 88(2):115-20.

116. Jallo GI, Danish S, Velasquez L: Intramedullary low-grade astrocytomas long-term outcome following radical surgery. JNeurooncol. 2001, 53:61-66.

117. Jallo GI, Freed D, Epstein F: Intramedullary spinal cord tumors in children.Childs Nerv Syst 2003, 19:641-649.

118. Jallo GI, Freed D, Zareck M, Epstein F: Clinical presentation and optimal management for intramedullary cavernous malformations. Neurosurg Focus. 2006, 21(1):e10.

119. Jallo GI, Kothbauer KF, Epstein FJ: Contact laser microsurgery. Childs Nerv Syst.
2002,18:333-336.

120. Jeffrey P B, Scott E: Spinal lipomas. Neurosurg Focus. 2001, 10 (1): Article 3.

121. Jellema K, van Overbeeke J J, Teepen L: Time to diagnosis of intraspinal tumors. European Journal of Neurology. 2005, 12/ 8, 621-624.

122. Jellinger K, Kothbauer P, Sunder-Plassman E: Intramedullary spinal cord metastases. J Neurol. 1979, 220: 31-41.

123. Jeong SM, Chung YG, Lee JB: Intracranial dissemination from spinal cord anaplastic astrocytoma. J Korean Neurosurg Soc. 2010, 47(1):68-70.

124. Jones SJ, Buonamassa S, Crockard HA: Two cases of quadriparesis following anterior cervical discectomy with normal perioperative somatosensory evoked potentials. J Neurol Neurosurg Psychiatry. 2003, 74/2:273-6.

125. Jyothirmayi R, Madhavan J, Nair MK, Rajan B: Conservative surgery and radiotherapy in the treatment of spinal cord astrocytoma. Journal of NeuroOncology. 1997,33: 205-211.

126. Kalayci M, Cagavi F, Gül S: Intramedullary spinal cord metastases: diagnosis and treatment-an illustrated review. Acta Neurochir. 2004, 146: 1347-1354.

127. Kawakami N, Mimatsu K, Kato F: Intraoperative sonography of intramedullary spinal cord tumors. Neuroradiology. 1992, 34:436-439.

128. Kawasakı K, Wakabayashi K, Koizumi T, Tanaka R, Takahashi H: Spinal cord involvement of primary central nervous system lymphomas: histopathological examination of 14 autopsy cases. Neuropathology. 2002, Mar; 22(1):13-8.

129. Keegan. BM, Flanagan E, O'Neill BP: Primary intramedullary spinal cord lymphoma. Neurology. 2011, 77:784-791.

130. Kharkar S, Shuck J, Conway J: The natural history of conservatively managed symptomatic intramedullary spinal cord cavernomas. Neurosurgery. 2007, 60: 865-872.

131. Kim CH, Wang KC, Kim SK: Spinal intramedullary lipoma report of three cases. Spinal Cord. 2003, 41:310-315.

132. Kim MS, Chung CK, Choe G, Kim IH: Intramedullary spinal cord astrocytoma in adults: postoperative outcome. J Neurooncol. 2001 Mar;52(1):85-

94.

133. Klekamp.J, Samii M: Surgery of Spinal Tumors Springer-Verlag Berlin Heidelberg. 2007, 120-14.

134. Koos WT, Day JD: Neurological surgery at the University of Vienna. Neurosurgery. 1996, 39:583-587.

135. Kopelson G, Linggood RM, Kleinman GM: Management of intramedullary Spinal cord tumors. Radiology. 1980, 135(2):473-9.

136. Koschorek F, Jensen HP, Terwey B: The dynamic evaluation of the cervical spinal canal and spinal cord by magnetic resonance imaging during movement. Acta Radiol Suppl. 1987, 369:727-9.

137. Kothbauer KF: Neurosurgical management of intramedullary spinal cord tumors in children. Pediatr Neurosurg 2007, 43(3):222-235.

138. Kothbauer KF: Motor Evoked Potential Monitoring for Intramedullary Spinal Cord Tumor Surgery Vedran Deletis Jay L. Shils Neurophysiology in Neurosurgery A Modern Intraoperative Approach Copyright, Elsevier Science (USA). 2002,73-89.

139. KrifaH: intramedullary tumors.http//pf mh.uvt.rnu.tn/id/eprint/194, 2011.

140. Kriss TC, Kriss VM: History of the operating microscope: From magnifying glass to microneurosurgery. Neurosurgery, 1998, 42:899-908.

141. Kucia EJ, Bambakidis NC, Chang SW, Spetzler RF: Surgical Technique and Outcomes in the Treatment of Spinal Cord Ependymomas,Part 1: Intramedullary Ependymomas. Neurosurgery. 2011,68[ONS Suppl 1]:ons57-ons63.

142. Kumar R, Singh V: Intramedullary mass lesion of the spinal cord in children of a developing milieu. PediatrNeurosurg. 2004, 40(1):16-22.

143. Labauge P, Bouly S, Parker F: Outcome in 53 patients with spinal cord cavernomas. SurgNeurol 2008, 70:176-181.

144. Lang J: Clinical Anatomy of the Cervical Spine. Thieme, Stuttgart (Georg Thieme Verlag, Stuttgart. 1993.

144 bis. Langeron O, Vivien B, Lille F: Monitorage peropératoire de la moelle épinière. Conférences d'actualisation 1997, p. 185-96. 1997 Elsevier, Paris, and SFAR.

145. Lazorthe.C, Couate A.Djindjin.R: Vascularisation et circulation de la moelle épinière anatomie physiologie, angiographie Masson et Cie Paris 1973, 1-286.

146. Lee DK, Choe WJ, Chung CK: Spinal cord hemangioblastoma: surgical strategy and clinical outcome. JNeurooncol. 2003, 61(1):27-34.

147. Lee J, Parsa AT, Ames CP, McCormick PC: Clinical management of intramedullary spinal ependymomas in adults. Neurosurg Clin N Am. 2006 Jan; 17(1):21-7.

148. Lee M, Epstein F, Rezai AR: Non neoplastic intramedullary spinal cord lesions mimicking tumors. Neurosurgery. 1998, 43:788-795.

149. Lin YH, Huang CI, Wong TT: Treatment of spinal cord ependymomas by surgery with or without postoperative radiotherapy. JNeurooncol 2005, 71/2:205-10.

150. Linstadt DE, Wara WM, Leibel SA: Postoperative radiotherapy of primary spinal cord tumors.Int J Radiat Oncol Biol Phys. 1989, 16:1397- 403.

151. Liu W, James CD, Frederick L: PTEN/MMAC1 mutations and EGFR amplification in glioblastomas. Cancer Res. 1997, 57:5254-5257.

152. Lonser RR, Weil RJ, Wanebo JE: Surgical management of spinal cord hemangioblastomas in patients with von Hippel-Lindau disease. J Neurosurg 2003, 98:106-116.

153. Louis DN, Ohgaki H, Wiestler OD: WHO Classification of Tumours of the Central Nervous System. 4th ed. Lyon: International Agency for Research on Cancer (IARC); 2007.

154. Lowe GM: Magnetic resonance imaging of intramedullary spinal cord tumors. J Neurooncol. 2000, 47:195-210.

155. Lu DC, Chou D, Mummaneni PV: A comparison of mini open and open approaches for resection of thoracolumbar intradural spinal tumors. J Neurosurg Spine. 2011 Jun; 14(6):758-64.

156. Lu DC, Lawton MT: Clinical presentation and surgical management of intramedullary spinal cord cavernous malformations. Neurosurg Focus. 2010, Sep; 29(3):E12.

157. Lunardi P, Licastro G, Missori P: A Management of intramedullary tumors in children. Acta Neurochir (Wien). 1993, 120:59-65.

158. Magni .C, Yapo .P, Sonier C.B: Primary intramedullary melanoma a propos d'un cas. Journal of Neuroradiology. 1996, 23/1 p. 41.

159. Maillot C: The perimedullary spaces, constitution, organization and relations with the cerebrospinal fluid. J radiol. 1990,71 :539-39.

160. Maiuri F, Iaconetta G, Gallicchio B: Intraoperative sonography for spinal tumors. Correlations with MR findings and surgery. J Neurosurg Sci. 2000, 44/3:115-22.

161. Mandigo CE, Ogden AT, Angevine PD: operative management of spinal hemangioblastoma Neurosurgery. 2009, 65:1166-1177.

162. Manelfe C, Lazorthe G, Roulleau J: arterioles de la dure mére rachidienne chez l'homme. acta radiol (diagn). 1972,13: 829-4.

163. Mansfield P: Multi- planar image formation using NMR spin echoes. J Phys C Solid State Phys. 1977, 10:L55-L58.

164. Matsyama Y, Sakai Y, Katayama Y, Imagama S, Ito Z: Surgical results of intramedullary spinal cord tumor with spinal cord monitoring to guide extent of resection. J Neurosurg Spine. 2009, May; 10 (5):404-13.

165. McCormick PC, Torres R, Post KD: Intramedullary ependymoma of the spinal cord. J Neurosurg. 1990, 72:523-532.

166. McGirt MJ, Chaichana KL, Atiba AS: Incidence of spinal deformity after resection of intra medullary spinal cord tumors in children who underwent laminectomy compared with laminoplasty. J Neurosurg Pediatr. 2008, Jan; 1(1):57-62.

167. McGirt MJ, Chaichana KL, Attenello F, Witham T, Bydon A, Yao KC, Jallo GI; Spinal deformity after resection of cervical intramedullary spinal cord tumors in children. Childs Nerv Syst. 2008, Jun; 24(6):735-9.

168. McGirt MJ, Constantini S, Jallo GI: Correlation of a preoperative grading scale with progressive spinal deformity following surgery for intramedullary spinal cord tumors in children. J Neurosurg Pediatr. 2008, Oct; 2(4): 277-81.

169. McGirt MJ, Goldstein IM, Chaichana KL, Tobias ME, Kothbauer KF, Jallo GI: Extent of surgical resection of malignant astrocytomas of the spinal cord: outcome analysis of 35 patients. Neurosurgery. 2008, Jul; 63(1): 55-60 ; discussion 60-1.

170. McLone DG, Naidich TP: Laser resection of fifty spinal lipomas. Neurosurgery. 1986, 18:611-615.

171. Mehta AI, Mohrhaus CA, Husain AM, Karikari IO, Hughes B, Hodges T: Dorsal Column Mapping for Intramedullary Spinal Cord Tumor Resection Decreases Dorsal Column Dysfunction. J Spinal Disord Tech. 2012, 25: 205209.

172. Mehta GU, Asthagiri AR, Bakhtian KD, Lonser RR: Functional outcome after resection of spinal cord hemangioblastomas associated with von Hippel-Lindau disease. J Neurosurg: Spine. 2010,12. 233- 242.

173. Mihara H, Kondo S, Takeguchi H: Spinal cord morphology and dynamics during cervical laminoplasty: evaluation with intraoperative sonography. Spine. 2007, 1; 32/21:2306-9.

174. Milano MT, Johnson MD, Sul J: Primary spinal cord glioma: a surveillance, epidemiology, and end results database study. J Neurooncol. 2010; 98:83-92.

175. Miller DJ, McCutcheon IE: Hemangioblastomas and other uncommon intramedullary tumors. J Neurooncol. 2000 May; 47(3):253-70.

176. Minehan KJ, Shaw EG, Scheithauer BW: Spinal cord astrocytoma: pathological and treatment considerations. J Neurosurg. 1995, 83: 590-595.

177. Mirone G, Cinalli G, Spennato P: Hydrocephalus and spinal cord tumors: a review. Childs Nerv Syst. 2011, Oct; 27(10):1741-9.

178. Miyazawa N, Hida K, Iwasaki Y: MRI at 1.5 T of intramedullary ependymoma and classification of pattern of contrast enhancement. Neuroradiology. 2000, 42:828-32.

179. Mora J,Cruz O, Gala S: Successful treatment of childhood intramedullary spinal cord astrocytomas with irinotecan and cisplatin. Neuro Oncol. 2007, Jan; 9(1): 39-46.

180. Mork SJ, Loken AC: Ependymoma: a follow-up study of 101 cases. Cancer. 1977, 40:907-915.

181. Nadkarni TD, Rekate HL: Pediatric intramedullary spinal cord tumors. Critical review of the literature. Childs Nerv Syst. 1999, 15:17-28.

182. Najjar MW, Kusske JA, Hasso AN: Dorsal intramedullary dermoids. Neurosurg. 2005, 8(4):320-5.

183. Nakamura M, Ishii K, Tsuji T, Takaishi H, Matsumoto M: Surgical treatment of intramedullary spinal cord tumors: prognosis and complications. Spinal Cord. 2008, Apr; 46(4):282-6.2

184. Nauta HJW, Dolan ED, Yasargil MG: Microsurgical anatomy of spinal subarachnoid space. Surg Neurol. 1983, 19:431-437.

184 bis. Netter.F H: Atlas of human anatomy. Elsevier Masson; Edition: 5th edition (July 6, 2011).

185. Nicholas DS, Weller RO: The fine anatomy of the human spinal meninges. A light and scanning electron microscopy study. J Neurosurg. 1988, 69:276-282.

186. Nieuwenhuys.R, Voogd.J, van Huijzen.C: The Human Central Nervous System. Springer Berlin Heidelberg Germany 4th Ed: 2008.

187. Nishikawa M, Ohata K, Ishibashi K: The anterolateral partial vertebrectomy approach for ventrally located cervical intramedullary cavernous angiomas. Neurosurgery. 2006, 59 (1 Suppl 1):ONS58-ONS63.

188. Norman D, Mills CM, Brant- Zawadzki M: Magnetic resonance imaging of the spinal cord and canal: Potentials and limitations. AJR Am J Roentgenol. 1983,

141:1147-1152.

189. Nuti C, Vassal F, Tourneux .H, Dumas: An observation of intramedullary neuroma. Revue de la littérature. Neurosurgery. 2007,53/ 5 - p. 437.

190. OgdenAT, FesslerRG: Minimally invasive Resection of intramedullary ependymoma: case report. Neurosurgery. 2009, Dec; 65(6):E1203-4.

191. Oh MC, Ivan ME, Sun MZ, Kaur G, Safaee M, ParsaAT: Adjuvant radiotherapy delays recurrence following subtotal resection of spinal cord ependymomas. Neuro Oncol. 2013, Feb; 15(2):208-15.

192. Ojemann RG, Crowell RM, Ogilvy CS: Management of cranial and spinal cavernous angiomas (honored guest lecture). Clin Neurosurg. 1993, 40:98-123.

193. Ortega-Martinez M, Cabezudo JM, Fernández-Portales I: Multiple filum terminale hemangioblastomas symptomatic during pregnancy.Case report. J Neurosurg Spine. 2007, 7:254-258.

194. Pallatroni HF, Hug EB, Ball PA: Atypical teratoid/rhabdoid tumor of the spine in an adult: case report and review of the literature. J Neurooncol. 2007, 84(1):49-55.

195. Park CH, Hyun SJ, Kim KJ: Spinal intramedullary ependymal cysts: a case report and review of the literature. J Korean Neurosurg Soc. 2012 Jul; 52(1):67-70.

196. Park DM, Zhuang Z, Chen L: von Hippel-Lindau disease-associated hemangioblastomas are derived from embryologic multipotent cells. PLo S Med. 2007, 4(2):e60.

197. Parsa AT: Intramedullary Spinal Cord Tumors: Molecular insights and Surgical Innovation Chapter 10, Intramedullary Spinal Cord Tumors: Molecular insights book 2. neurosurgeon.org. Biol. 2004, 15:171-176.

198. Parsons R: Human cancer, PTEN and the PI-3 kinase pathway. Semin Cell Dev Biol. 2004, 15(2):171-6.

199. Patil CG, Patil TS, Lad SP, Boakye M: Complications and outcomes after spinal cord tumor resection in the United States from 1993 to 2002. Spinal Cord. 2008, May; 46(5):375-9.

200. Patronas NJ, Courcoutsakis N, Bromley CM: Intramedullary and spinal canal tumors in patients with neurofibromatosis 2: MR imaging findings and correlation with genotype. Radiology. 2001, 218:434-442.

201. Peker S, Ozgen S, Ozek MM: Surgical treatment of intramedullary spinal cord ependymomas. Can outcome be predicted by tumor parameters? J Spinal Disord Tech. 2004, 17:51-521.

202. Peng L, Qi ST, Chen Z, Fen WF: Radical microsurgical treatement of intramedullary spinal cord. Chin Med J (Eng). 2006 Aug 20; 119 (16): 1343-7

203. Pietila TA, Stendel R, Schilling A: Surgical treatment of spinal hemangioblastomas. Acta Neurochir (Wien). 2000, 142:879-886.

204. Quinones-Hinojosa A, Gulati M, Lyon R: spinal cord mapping as an adjunct for resection of intramedullary tumors: surgical technique with case illustrations. Neurosurgery. 2002, 51:1199-1207.

205. Rabieshang.P, Paleirac R, michel f Note on the development and organization of medullary meningeal spaces. CR ass anat. 1962,119 :1122-33.

206. Raco A, Esposito V, Lenzi J: long-term follow-up of intramedullary spinal cord tumors: a series of 202 cases. Neurosurgery 2005, 56:972-981.

207. Raco A, Piccirilli M, Landi A: High-grade intramedullary astrocytomas: 30 years experience at the Neurosurgery Department of the University of Rome "Sapienza". J Neurosurg Spine 2010, 12:144-153.

208. Rajshekhar V, Velayutham P, Joseph M, Babu KS: Factors predicting the feasibility of monitoring lower-limb muscle motor evoked potentials in patients undergoing excision of spinal cord tumors. J Neurosurg Spine. 2011 Jun; 14(6):748-53.

209. Regelsberger J, Fritzsche E, Langer N, Westphal M: Intraoperative sonography of intra- and extramedullary tumors. Ultrasound Med Biol. 2005 May; 31(5):593-8.

210. Reid MH: Ultrasonic visualization of a cervical cord cystic astrocytoma. AJR Am J Roentgenol 1978, 131/5:907-8.

211. Rennels ML, Gregory TF, Blaumanis OR: Evidence for a paravascular fluid circulation in the mammalian central nervous system, provided by the rapid distribution of tracer protein throughout the brain from the subarachnoid space. Brain Res 1985, 4; 326(1):47-63.

212. Richard A. Prayson, Karl M: Central Nervous System, Frozen Section Library 6, Springer Science+Business Media, LLC 2011, 55-78.

213. Robertson DP, Kirkpatrick JB, Harper RL, Mawad ME: Spinal intramedullary ependymal cyst. Report of three cases. J Neurosurg 1991, 75:312-316.

214. Rodrigues GB, Waldron JN, Wong S: A retrospective analysis of 52 cases of spinal cord glioma managed with radiation therapy. Int J Radiat Oncol Biol Phys 2000, 48,837-842.

215. Rosomoff HL, Carroll F: Reaction of neoplasm and brain to laser. Arch Neurol 1966, 14:143-148.

216. Roux FX. Rey A. George B: Adult intramedullary astrocytomas and ependymomas: Does therapeutic tactic influence long-term outcome? Review of 23 operated cases and discussion of the literature. Neurosurgery 1984,30:99-105.

217. Rubinstein LJ: Tumors of the Central Nervous System, fasc 6, Washington in Armed Forces Institute of Pathology (ed): Atlas of Tumors Pathology 1972, pp 19-126.

218. Ryu SI. Kim DH. Chang SD: Stereotactic radiosurgery for hemangiomas and ependymomas of the spinal cord. Neurosurg Focus 15: Article 10, 2003.

219. Saito K, Morita A, Shibahara J, Kirino T: Spinal intramedullary ependymal cyst; a case report and review of the literature. Acta Neurochir (Wien). 2005 Apr; 147(4):443-6.

220. Sakuma S, Iwasaki Y, Isu T: A case of intramedullary spinal cord metastasis from adenocarcinoma of corpus uteri. No Shinkei Geka Japan 1990, 18:653-657.

221. Sala F, Bricolo A, Faccioli F: Surgery for intramedullary spinal cord tumors: the role of intraoperative (neurophysiological) monitoring. Euro Spine J 2007, 16 (Suppl 2):S130-S139.

222. Sala F, Palandri G, Deletis V: Motor evoked potential monitoring improves outcome after surgery for intramedullary spinal cord tumors: a historical control study. Neurosurgery 2006, 58:1129-1143.

223. Sami M, Klekamp J: Surgical results of 100 intramedullary tumors in relation to accompanying syringomyelia. Neurosurgery 1994, 35:865-873.

224. Sandalcioglu IE, Wiedemayer H, Gasser T: Intramedullary spinal cord cavernous malformations: clinical features and risk of hemorrhage. Neurosurg 2003, 26: 253-256.

225. Sandler HM, Papadopoulos SM, Thornton AF Jr: Spinal Cord Astrocytomas: Results of Therapy. Neurosurgery 1992, 31(6):1136.

226. Sattar MT, Bannister CM, Turnbull I W: occult spinal dysraphism the common combination of lesions and the clinical manifestations in 50 patients. Eur J Pediatr Surg 1996, 6 Suppl 1:10-14.

227. Scheinemann K, Bartels U, Huang A: Survival and functional outcome of childhood spinal cord low-grade gliomas. J Neurosurg Pediatrics 2009, 4:254-261.

228. Schwartz TH, McCormick PC: Intramedullary ependymomas: clinical presentation, surgical treatment strategies and prognosis. J Neurooncol 2000, 47:211-218.

229. Sciubba DM, Liang D, Kothbauer KF: the evolution of intra medullary spinal cord tumors surgery. Neurosurgery 2009, 65[ONS Suppl 1]:ons84 -ons92.

230. Seo HS, Kim JH, Lee DH: Nonenhancing intramedullary astrocytomas and other MR imaging features: a retrospective study and systematic review. AJNR Am J Neuroradiol 2010, 31(3):498-503.

231. Setzer M, Murtagh RD, Murtagh FR, Eleraky M, Jain S: Diffusion tensor imaging tractography in patients with intramedullary tumors: comparison with intraoperative findings and value for prediction of tumor respectability. J Neurosurg Spine 2010, 13:371-38.

232. Sgouros S, Malluci CL, Jackowski A: Spinal ependymomas the value of postoperative radiotherapy for residual disease control. Br J Neurosurg 1996, 10:559-566.

233. Sharma GK, Kucia EJ, Spetzler RF: Spontaneous intramedullary hemorrhage of spinal hemangioblastoma: case report. Neurosurgery 2009, 65(3):E627-628.

234. Sharma M, Mally R, Velho V: Ruptured conus medullaris dermoid cyst with fat droplets in the central. Asian Spine J. 2013 Mar; 7(1):50-4.

235. Shin DA, Kim SH, Kim KN, Shin HC, Yoon DH: Surgical management of spinal cord haemangioblastoma. Acta Neurochir (Wien). 2008 Mar; 150(3):215-20.

236. Shirato H, Kamada T, Hida K, Koyanagi I: The role of radiotherapy in the management of spinal cord glioma. Int J Radiat Oncol Biol Phys 1995, 33: 323-328.

237. Shrivastava RK, Epstein FJ, Perin NI: Intramedullary spinal cord tumors in patients older than 50 years of age: management and outcome analysis. J Neurosurg Spine 2005, 2:249-255.

238. Sigal R, Denys A, Halimi P, Shapeero L, Doyon D,Boudghene F: Ventriculus terminalis of the conus medullaris: MR imaging in four patients with congenital dilatation. AJNR Am J Neuroradiol 1991, 12:733-737.

239. Simon SL, Auerbach JD, Garg S, Sutton LN: Efficacy of spinal instrumentation and fusion in the prevention of post laminectomy spinal deformity in children with intramedullary spinal cord tumors. J Pediatr Orthop 2008 Mar; 28(2):244-9.

240. Slooff JL, Kernohan JW, MacCarty CS: Primary intramedullary tumors of the spinal cord and filum terminal. Philadelphia: WB Saunders Company, 1964.

241. Solomon RA, Stein BM: Unusual spinal cord enlargement related to intramedullary hemangioblastoma. J Neurosurg 1988, 68: 550-553.

242. Stabouli S, Sdougka M, Tsitspoulos P: Primary atypical teratoid/rhabdoid tumor of the spine in an infant. Hippokratia 2010, 14(4): 286-288.

243. Stebbins CE, Kaelin WG, Pavletich NP: Structure of the VHL-ElonginC ElonginB complex: implications for VHL tumor suppressor function. Science 1999, 284: 455-461.

244. Steiger HJ, Turowski B, Hanggi D: Prognostic factors for the outcome of surgical and conservative treatment of symptomatic spinal cord cavernous malformation: a review of a series of 20 patients. Neurosurg Focus. 2010 Sep; 29(3):E13.

245. Stein BM, McCormick PC: Intramedullary neoplasms and vascular malformations. Clin Neurosurg 1992, 39:361-387.

246. Sun B, Wang C, Wang J: MRI: features of intramedullary spinal cord ependymomas. J Neuroimaging 2003, 13:346-51.

247. Takahashi I, IwasakiY, HidaK: Clinical study of intraspinal neoplasms in children. No Shinkei Geka 1996, 24:605-611.

248. Takenaka N, Imanishi T, Kondoh A: Primary intramedullary melanocytoma of the medulla oblongata: a case report. Shinkei Geka 1996, 24:247-252.

249. Taricco MA, Guirado VM, Fontes RB: Surgical treatment of primary intramedullary spinal cord tumors in adult patients. Arq Neuropsiquiatr 2008, 66(1):59-63.

250. Tekautz TM, Fuller CE, Blaney S: Atypical teratoid/rhabdoid tumors (ATRT): improved survival in children 3 years of age and older with radiation therapy and high-dose alkylator-based chemotherapy. J Clin Oncol 2005,23:1491-1499.

251. Timothy E.G. Hassall, Anne E. Mitchell: Carboplatin chemotherapy for progressive intramedullary spinal cord low-gradegliomas in children: Three case studies and a review of the literature. Neuro-Oncology 2001 October, PP251-257n.

252. Turnbull IM, Brieg A, Hassler O: Blood supply of cervical spinal cord in man: A microangiographic cadaver study. J Neurosurg 1966, 24:951-965.

253. Van Velthoven V, Reinacher PC, Klisch J: Treatment of intramdedullary hemangioblastomas, with special attention to Von Hippel-Lindau disease. Neurosurgery 2003, 53:1306-1314 /336.

254. Vincent Di Marino, Yves Etienne: Color photographic atlas of the central nervous system. Springer-Verlag France, Paris, 2011, 79-93.

255. Vishteh AG, Sankhla S, Anson JA: Surgical resection of intramedullary spinal cord cavernous malformations: delayed complications, long-term outcomes, and association with cryptic venous malformations. Neurosurgery 1997, 41:1094-1101.

256. Von Deimling A, Louis DN, Wiestler OD: Molecular pathways in the formation of gliomas. Glia 1995, 15:328-338.

257. Von Haken MS, White EC, Daneshvar-Shyesther L: Molecular genetic analysis of chromosome arm 17p and chromosome arm 22q DNA sequences in sporadic pediatric ependymomas. Genes Chromosomes. Cancer 1996, 17:37-44.

258. Vortmeyer AO, Gnarra JR, Emmert-Buck MR: Von Hippel-Lindau gene deletion detected in the stromal cell component of a cerebellar hemangioblastoma associated with von Hippel-Lindau disease. Hum Pathol 1997, 28:540-543.

259. Wahab SH, Simpson JR, Michalski JM: Long term outcome with post-operative radiation therapy for spinal canal ependymoma. J Neurooncol 2007, 83(1):85-89.

260. Watanabe M, Nomura T, Toh E, Sato M, Mochida J: Intramedullary Spinal Cord Metastasis A Clinical and Imaging Study of Seven Patients. J Spinal Disord Tech
2006,19:43-47.

261. White JB, Miller GM, Layton KF, Krauss WE: Nonenhancing tumors of the spinal cord. J Neurosurg Spine. 2007 Oct; 7(4):403-7.

262. Wood EH, Berne AS, Taveras JM: The value of radiation therapy in the management of intrinsic tumors of the spinal cord. Radiology. 1954 Jul; 63(1):11-24.

263. Woodworth GF, Chaichana KL, McGirt MJ, Sciubba DM, Jallo GI, Gokaslan Z, Wolinsky JP, Witham TF: Predictors of ambulatory function after surgical resection of intramedullary spinal cord tumors. Neurosurgery. 2007 Jul; 61(1):99-105.

264. Wu PS, Yao WJ: F-18 FDG PET in Spinal Cord Pilocytic Astrocytoma. Clin Nucl Med 2010, 35: 649-650.

265. Yang S, Yang X, Hong G: Surgical Treatment of One Hundred Seventy-Four Intramedullary Spinal Cord Tumors. Spine 2009, 34/24, pp 2705-2710.

266. Yao K, Kothbauer KF, Bitan F,Constantini S, Epstein FJ, Jallo GI: Spinal deformity and intramedullary tumor surgery. Childs Nerv Syst 2000, 16:530.

267. Yao KC, McGirt MJ, Chaichana KL, Constantini S, Jallo GI: Risk factors for progressive spinal deformity following resection of intramedullary spinal cord tumors in children: an analysis of 161 consecutive cases. J Neurosurg 2007, Dec; 107 (6 Suppl):463-8.

268. Yasargil MG, Antic J, Laciga R: The microsurgical removal of intramedullary spinal hemangioblastomas. Report of twelve cases and a review of the literature. SurgNeurol 1976, 3:141-148.

269. Yoshino M, Morita A, Shibahara J, Kirino T: Radiation-induced spinal cord cavernous malformation. Case report. JNeurosurg 2005; 102(Suppl 1):101-104.

270. Zentner J, Hassler W, Gawehn J: Intramedullary cavernous angiomas. Surg Neurol 1989, 31:64-68.

271. Zhou H, Miller D, Schulte DM, Benes L: Intraoperative ultrasound assistance in treatment of intradural spinal tumours. Clin Neurol Neurosurg. 2011 Sep; 113(7):531-7.

272. Zileli M, Coskun E, Ozdamar N: Surgery of intramedullary spinal cord tumors. Eur Spine J 1996, 5:243-250.

273. Zentner J, Hassler W, Gawehn J: Intramedullary cavernous angiomas. Surg Neurol 1989, 31:64-68.

LIST OF FIGURES

Fig.40: Pre- and postoperative MRI and operative view of a dermoid cyst with leakage of lipid droplets into the ependymal canal after excision. Right: operative view.
Fig.41: T1 MRI with gadolinium: T9-T10 intramedullary melanocytoma, homogeneously enhanced.
Fig.42: Sagittal MRI T2, T1 and operative view of an ependymo-glial cyst of the terminal cone.
Right: operative view.

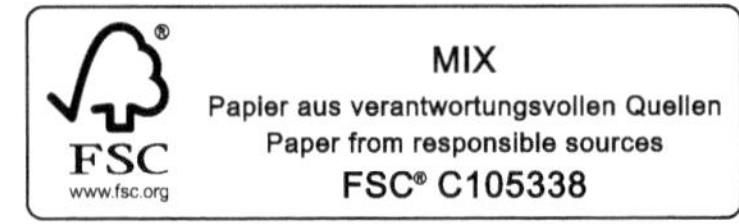

Printed by Books on Demand GmbH, Norderstedt / Germany